STO

**DO NOT REMOVE
CARDS FROM POCKET**

2·83

Prevent Your Heart Attack

Prevent Your Heart Attack

NORMAN M. KAPLAN, M. D.

CHARLES SCRIBNER'S SONS
NEW YORK

Copyright © 1982 Norman M. Kaplan

Library of Congress Cataloging in Publication Data

Kaplan, Norman M., 1931–
    Prevent your heart attack.

    Bibliography: p.
    Includes index.
    1. Heart—Infarction—Prevention.   I. Title.
RC685.I6K34   1983   616.1′205   82-16853
ISBN 0-684-17797-8

1 3 5 7 9 11 13 15 17 19   F/C   20 18 16 14 12 10 8 6 4 2

Printed in the United States of America.

Contents

Introduction

Most likely, you and I will die of a cardiovascular event, either a heart attack or a stroke. If the event occurs suddenly, at age 70 or 75, it may be a quick, relatively painless death. Compared with the prolonged miseries of cancer, we are certainly much less concerned about heart and vascular disease. Each year we contribute almost twice as much to the Cancer Society as we do to the American Heart Association.

But cardiovascular disease does not attack the elderly alone. It is the most common cause of death for those 40 to 60 years old as well. And both heart attacks and strokes disable hundreds of thousands of active, productive people each year, adding billions of dollars of expense and seemingly endless days of suffering and misery to their lives.

This book is offered as a practical, commonsense guide to help decrease the chances of having cardiovascular disease. It has been written with these beliefs in mind:

- You are, in large measure, responsible for your own health.
- If aware of the consequences, you can stop unhealthy practices and, if they are not offered in too drastic or abrupt a manner, you will adopt healthier habits.

- By changing relatively few habits, you can decrease your chances of having cardiovascular disease.

This book is neither the first nor the last to be written on the prevention of heart disease. But most that I have seen—and I've looked at virtually every one written in the United States over the past ten years—suffer from one of two defects: they are full of misleading, oversimplified gimmicks, promising too much, too fast; or they are too detailed, too long and complicated, making it difficult for most readers to use their advice.

So this book is short, to the point, and, I hope, easy to read and follow. But at the same time it is accurate and up-to-date. It asks no more than you should be able to perform and to deliver. Each of the risks for cardiovascular disease is examined closely, and practical, medically proven advice is provided for you to use in reducing your risks, not as short-term abrupt reversals of habit but as gradual, long-lasting changes.

Such changes will help. When the everyday health and life-style practices of almost seven thousand adults in Alameda County, California, were examined, they were found to relate strongly to their physical well-being. These practices were: sleeping seven to eight hours, eating breakfast regularly, not eating between meals, keeping a desirable weight, exercising regularly, drinking alcohol in moderation, and not smoking cigarettes. At every age, the more of these practices followed, the better the physical status. Though cardiovascular health was not specifically examined, I can assure you that it went along with the overall health status.

Before starting the specifics, one more generality: everyone is preaching "do-it-yourself," "self-care," "take individual responsibility." Part of this new interest in putting more responsibility for our health on ourselves comes from repeated claims—almost all unsubstantiated—that the medical profession is "harmful to your health." Part comes from the awareness that the costs of medical care, aimed at cure, are outstripping our ability or at least our willingness to pay for them.

Another part comes from the realization that much—even most—of our current ill health is caused directly by our own bad habits: smoking, drinking, overeating, exercising too little, and constantly trying to do too much in too short a time.

It is becoming clear that we can *prevent* disease and live longer if we practice better health habits. That is the primary message of this book. But lest we become overwhelmed by this responsibility, let's remember that society at large, acting through our governments, must also be involved. Some people can't care for themselves. None of us has complete control over his life. The individual alone cannot provide the support for research to find the causes of and cures for diseases. A humane, sensible approach to the problem is for our institutions to provide the knowledge and the direction for self-care, to remove as many harmful things in our environment as possible, and to support those services that only society, through our governments, can supply.

My thanks to the many people who have provided the knowledge upon which this book is based—and to my wife, family, and friends who have given me the time and support to put it together.

ONE

Where We Are Today: The Latest Epidemic

For the last fifty years, cardiovascular disease has been the most common cause of death in the United States, killing almost 1 million Americans each year. It has been responsible for over half of all mortality; all other causes of death added together—cancer, accidents, pneumonia, diabetes, and other diseases—claim fewer victims than does cardiovascular disease. Similar statistics apply to other industrialized societies worldwide, though as we shall see there are considerable differences among various countries.

Notice the dark portion of the bars in Figure 1, representing the more than 200,000 deaths occurring each year among people under age 65. Cardiovascular disease is the number one cause of mortality.

Beyond the premature deaths, cardiovascular diseases afflict and incapacitate many people at their most productive time of life. Each year, over 500,000 Americans under age 65 have a heart attack and over 100,000 a stroke. Some can overcome these events: both Dwight Eisenhower and Lyndon Johnson performed the duties of what must be the most stress-filled job in the world after having a heart attack. Certainly, many who have a cardiovascular event can return to an active and productive life. But for most, life is shortened.

1

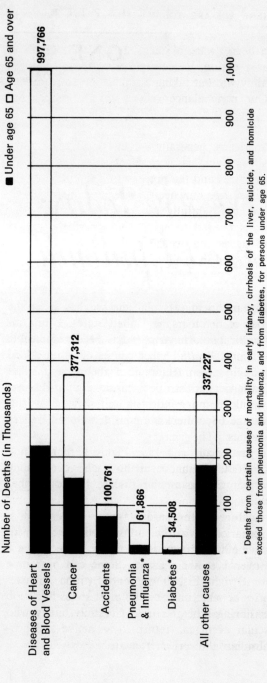

Number of Deaths (in Thousands)

■ Under age 65   □ Age 65 and over

997,766

377,312

100,761

61,866

34,508

337,227

Diseases of Heart and Blood Vessels

Cancer

Accidents

Pneumonia & Influenza*

Diabetes*

All other causes

100   200   300   400   500   600   700   800   900   1,000

* Deaths from certain causes of mortality in early infancy, cirrhosis of the liver, suicide, and homicide exceed those from pneumonia and influenza, and from diabetes, for persons under age 65.

Figure 1. Leading causes of death in the United States in 1976. Each bar represents the total number of deaths with the dark portion showing mortality of people under age 65. (Source: National Center for Health Statistics, U.S. Public Health Service)

You may have been aware of these statistics. But both as individuals and as a nation, we seem to accept them without concern and certainly without taking adequate action to reduce the death toll. Our nonchalance reflects several misconceptions:

- We Americans generally believe our high standard of living is accompanied by good health practices and the promise of a long life.
- We assume that our health care system—of which we are rightfully proud—will provide whatever is needed to ensure our health.
- Many of us assume we are doing as well as can be expected in avoiding the risks for heart disease.

Perhaps the most pertinent excuse is the impersonal nature of statistics. They concern others, not ourselves. But Dr. John Farquhar, in his book *The American Way of Life Need Not Be Hazardous to Your Health,* has projected these statistics onto a more dynamic screen. He divided the yearly toll of premature heart disease and stroke into a daily figure and then asked what would be our reaction if *each day of the year* 501 people, under age 65, were killed and 1562 were injured in jet airplane crashes. The answer is obvious. The public outcry would be immediate and loud. Congress, the FAA, and everyone else would demand action. All planes would be grounded until corrective measures were taken. Despite a great disruption of our transportation system, we would insist that no more deaths or disability occur from jumbo jet crashes.

Contrast that scenario to what we're now doing about those five hundred who die and fifteen hundred who are disabled *every day* from premature cardiovascular disease:

- Our personal habits continue to engender more hypertension, obesity, and high cholesterol levels.
- We subsidize the growing of tobacco with

public funds while cutting back on support of medical research.
- We continue to entice young people to smoke by having attractive models advertise cigarettes.
- We spend over 5 billion dollars a year promoting foods that are rich in calories, full of saturated fat, and heavily salted, while spending a pittance on nutritional education.
- More and more, our only exercise is turning on the TV set or manipulating a computer game.

Let us agree that the statistics document a serious problem that is not being adequately addressed. But behind them, another fact remains largely hidden: *most of the current premature disability and death can be prevented.* Though this may astonish you, there are two main bases for this statement. First, the relative frequency of cardiovascular disease has been steadily increasing, for as long as accurate vital statistics have been collected (Figure 2). It is clear that we have been doing things that are harmful to our cardiovascular health, because our genetic inheritance hasn't changed that much. According to the graph, the upward spiral really took off around 1920, though more for men than for women.

The argument has been made that the sharply rising curve—representing many millions of deaths—reflects the advent of easily affordable mechanical transportation. Henry Ford's Model T made it possible for us to ride not only to distant jobs but also to nearby grocery stores. Think of the difference between life today and when we had to walk or travel in horse-drawn carriages: most people worked in or near home, in cottage industries, and schools and shops were in the neighborhood. But with the automobile, jobs could be concentrated in far-off plants, and suburban shops and high rises could draw us from considerable distances. And with the accessibility of private and public transportation, walking almost anywhere soon became outmoded.

Rates per 100,000

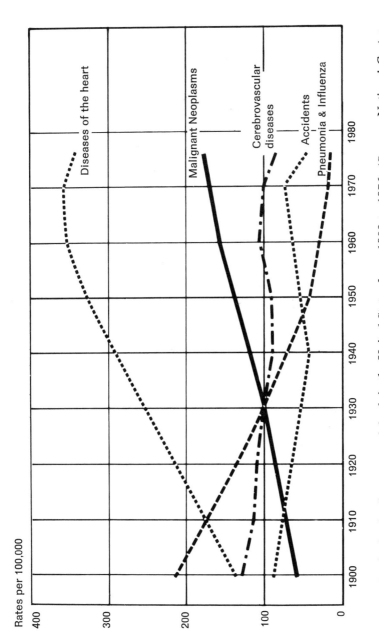

Figure 2. The five leading causes of death in the United States from 1900 to 1976. (Source: National Center for Health Statistics, U.S. Public Health Service)

Even beyond the obvious change in the levels of physical activity, there were many other changes brought on by advances in transportation and other areas of twentieth-century mechanization. Work increasingly became concentrated in more structured and stressful environments. Food no longer needed to be grown close by, so that it could be eaten before it spoiled; instead, it could be processed, frozen or canned, resulting in a longer shelf life but also including a host of potentially harmful additives, not the least of which is a large quantity of table salt. For many reasons, more women left working in the kitchen for other activities, so that convenience foods and fast-food outlets sprouted in profusion. Consider also the environmental pollution engendered by the automobile.

But let's not lay too much blame on Henry Ford and his successors. Many others have to share in it. We certainly can't forget the founders of the American tobacco industry, Buck Duke and R. J. Reynolds, who, with the help of Madison Avenue, convinced over 50 million Americans that it was better to "reach for a Lucky instead of a sweet."

We'll consider cigarettes, and salt, and other probable causes of our present situation in subsequent chapters. But look again at the upper right corner of Figure 2. Note that the mortality curve for heart disease flattened about 1960 and actually has come down since the late '60s. This seemingly small break in the curve is really quite significant. It gives us the second major piece of evidence that cardiovascular disease is preventable.

Compare the rate of death from cardiovascular disease with that from other causes from 1960 on (Figure 3). Though there has been a slight decrease in noncardiovascular deaths, the graph shows a much steeper fall in mortality from cardiovascular diseases. This decrease first occurred in 1968 and has persisted in every year except 1980, when a slight rise was noted. This reflects a 20 to 40 percent decrease in deaths from both heart attacks and strokes, the statistics varying between men and women of different ages and races: the lives of as many as 1 million Americans have been saved. As a result, average life expectancy has jumped almost four years, the largest jump ever recorded for the adult population in the United States.

As you can imagine, there's been a great deal of interest in explaining what has happened. Everyone involved in health care would like to take credit for the improvement. And if we could discover the reason, maybe we could do even more to reduce the death rate further.

One possibility is that we are caring better for those already afflicted. Certainly, the increasing availability of intensive-care units, cardiopulmonary-resuscitation training, advanced life-support stations, new drugs, coronary bypass surgery, and many more technological advances have improved the chances for survival after a heart attack or stroke. But for most victims, these technologies are only a Band-Aid. The majority of patients

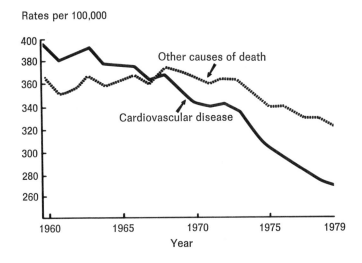

Figure 3. The death rates for cardiovascular diseases and all other causes of death in the U.S. from 1960 to 1979. (Source: National Center for Health Statistics, U.S. Public Health Service)

7

discharged from an intensive-care unit succumb to their underlying disease within the next year. Though both treatment and
bypass surgery have recently been shown to prolong life for
those who have severe heart disease, we must realize that for
most the relief is only temporary. There's really very little
evidence that existing cardiovascular disease can be *cured* with
any currently available therapy. And most of these advances
have been used for too short a time on too few patients to
explain what has happened since 1968.

The other possibility—and the more hopeful one—is that
we've reduced the actual development of cardiovascular disease. Though the evidence is only fragmentary, the number of
events, both heart attacks and strokes per unit of population,
has been shown to have decreased recently. However, it is very
difficult to measure accurately the number of these events.
Whereas the number of deaths (mortality) can be accurately
counted, being an incontrovertible and officially recorded occurrence, the number of disease events (morbidity) is much
less certain and not as well reported.

But surveys among carefully monitored populations have
shown a decrease in events. Perhaps the best survey comes
from investigators at the Mayo Clinic, where a complete record
of the health status of the residents of Rochester, Minnesota,
has been kept for many years. They have reported a significant
fall in the annual rate of occurrence (incidence) of both heart
attacks and strokes.

These and other statistics strongly support the view that
fewer Americans are dying from heart attacks and strokes,
because fewer are being stricken by these catastrophes. How
much better off we are, as individuals and as a society, to have
fewer of these incidents, so that we may cut back on the
ever-more costly and difficult rehabilitation of those afflicted
by them.

An ounce of prevention is worth far more than a pound of
cure, particularly when cure is usually only temporary relief.
Prevention is what this book is about. We have started the
process—that's the good news—but don't forget that despite

the dramatic fall in the incidence of cardiovascular mortality it remains our most common cause of death.

If we accept the evidence that less cardiovascular disease is occurring, the next obvious question is, What is responsible for the decrease? In the next chapter we will examine the factors that are the likely causes for the development of heart disease. Three will be shown to be the "major" culprits—high blood pressure, high blood cholesterol, and cigarette smoking. The severity and frequency of all three of these have been reduced over the past twenty years, preceding and likely being responsible for the falling rate of cardiovascular disease and death. The statistics show that

- Whereas only one in eight Americans with high blood pressure was being adequately treated in 1960, in some communities today as many as three in four have the disease under good control.
- The average level of blood cholesterol has fallen by some 15 milligrams per deciliter, reflecting a marked decrease in our consumption of butter, eggs, and animal fats.
- The consumption of tobacco products has fallen by over 20 percent and at least 15 million Americans have quit smoking cigarettes.

Other changes may also be partly responsible. Millions of Americans are running and jogging, with the hope that some good must surely come from all their effort. We have embraced a host of relaxation techniques, with hopes of relieving the effects of the stresses in our lives. We continue to embrace a new diet fad every six months, which at least enriches the purveyors of weight control by at least 5 billion dollars a year. At this point, let's simply say we have no proof that any of these have contributed to the fall in heart disease. Certainly, we've not controlled obesity: the average weight of American adults increased significantly from 1970 to 1980.

But many factors are probably involved. We will examine each in greater detail in this book. For now, the fact that we have made a beginning in reducing the toll is further proof that the problem is of our own making and—even more important—one that we *can overcome.*

Demographers have estimated that man's life expectancy in a modern, advanced society should be about 85 years. Though some may subscribe to the Biblical goal of 120, 4-score-and-5 is probably a more realistic reckoning. This estimate is based upon the longevity of groups of people whose healthy lifestyles and isolation from pollutants and other environmental stresses have protected them, as well as on laboratory studies on animals and human cells grown in test tubes.

In 1982, Americans had an overall life expectancy of about 71 years for men and 78 years for women. Thus, we're looking for an additional ten to fifteen years of life. But beyond longer life, we should be aiming for healthier life, free of the pain and disability of disease.

Are these goals reasonable? The fact that we've reduced deaths from heart disease over the last fifteen years by about 2 percent each year certainly is a strong indication of what can be accomplished. Even without knowing why we're doing better, a continued reduction will help.

But we have removed only the most accessible part of our problem; left behind is the hard core of those environmental and personal factors that are mainly responsible for cardiovascular disease. Many, if not most, of the more than 15 million Americans who have quit smoking were the casual, non-addicted, cocktail-party type of smoker. Whereas most hypertensives in some communities have been brought under good control, many millions have escaped intensive screening programs and even more resist the lifelong use of medication that produces improvement in their health, even though not obvious to the hypertensive. And, whereas many have switched from butter to margarine and from eggs to cereal, how many are willing to give up those juicy, delicious, marbled steaks—or, perhaps more to the point, those fat- and salt-filled hot dogs, hamburgers, and Kentucky-fried chicken?

Thus, our past accomplishments may not necessarily presage future success. We have a large reservoir of poor health practices that need to be improved. Our efforts may need to be more intensive, but with what we know today, a great amount of heart disease can be prevented. Two medical researchers, Drs. Gori and Richter, recently estimated that at least 39 percent and as many as 77 percent of the deaths now caused by cardiovascular disease are potentially preventable, based upon experience in other industrialized countries.

This book will show you how we can prevent a large amount of cardiovascular disease. First, we'll look at what is meant by cardiovascular disease—just what is involved in a heart attack or stroke. Then, we'll consider the puzzle of causation: the multiple factors which interact to produce cardiovascular disease. Each of the important, individual risk factors will be analyzed and practical strategies offered that will help remove or at least reduce that risk.

The advice will be usable, if you are willing to use it. I don't advocate extreme measures: the Pritikin program will almost certainly work, but I'm just as certain that you won't follow it. Similarly, I won't advise you to become a regular jogger, though if you're able and willing to jog regularly, it probably would help. On the other hand, I will advise you to stay away from such crazy gimmicks as the current fad in weight reduction, the Beverly Hills Diet.

Throughout the book, one overriding principle will be followed: none of the recommendations will do you any harm. As a physician, I am well aware of some of the harmful practices prescribed for the public with the best of intentions— worthless X-ray treatments for infants' normal thymus glands, ineffectual hormones to prevent abortions, unproven drugs to lower cholesterol levels: all three of these, offered in the hope of prevention, were subsequently found to increase the likelihood of cancer. The programs described in this book have been proven effective and safe by many years of use by millions of people.

TWO

The Puzzle of Heart Disease

Only recently have we recognized cardiovascular disease as our major public health problem. Various infectious diseases, particularly pneumonia and influenza, were the leading causes of death in the early 1900s. After improved sanitation, immunizations, and antibiotics reduced the impact of infections, more and more people lived long enough for cardiovascular diseases to become manifest. Though the hearts of Egyptian mummies who died over two thousand years ago were found to have been afflicted, more frequent and more extensive cardiovascular damage has been observed in recent years. Before considering the likely causes of this increase, let us clarify just what is meant by the terms we will use.

CIRCULATION IN THE NORMAL HEART

Quite simply, your heart is a muscular pump with two separate cylinders, each pushing about two ounces of blood through your lungs and body each time it contracts or beats (Figure 4). The blood is carried in a series of tubes which first become progressively smaller to deliver blood throughout the body and then enlarge again to return it to the heart. Thick-walled

12

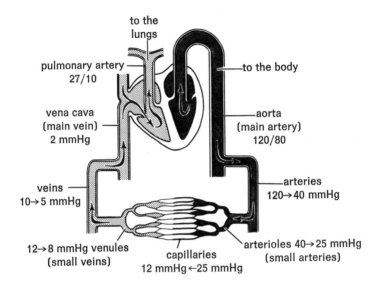

to the
lungs

pulmonary artery
27/10

vena cava
(main vein)
2 mmHg

veins
10→5 mmHg

12→8 mmHg venules
(small veins)

to the body

aorta
(main artery)
120/80

arteries
120→40 mmHg

arterioles 40→25 mmHg
(small arteries)

capillaries
12 mmHg←25 mmHg

Figure 4. A schematized view of the human heart and blood vessels showing blood pressures in various parts of the circulation.

arteries take the blood into the various organs of your body; microscopic *capillaries* allow the blood to transfer oxygen, glucose, and other essential nutrients to the cells of the various organs; thin-walled *veins* drain the blood and return it to the heart.

As shown in the lighter shading at the left side of Figure 4, the blood returning to the right side of the heart, emptied of much of its oxygen, is first pumped into the lungs. There oxygen is transferred into the red blood cells (corpuscles)

13

from the air inhaled during each breath. At the same time, carbon dioxide and other waste gases are released from the blood into the air in the lungs. That air is then exhaled.

The oxygen-enriched blood, shown in the darker shading at the right of Figure 4, returns to the left side of the heart. From there, it is pumped out into the main artery, the aorta, and then through the progressively smaller branches into the rest of the body.

Notice the numbers below each section of the circulation shown in Figure 4. They represent the normal levels of pressure within each section, measured as the height in millimeters (mm) that the pressure of blood would push a column of mercury (Hg) up a tube connected to the blood vessel. By the end of each heartbeat, referred to as *systole,* the heavily muscled left side of the heart engenders the highest level of pressure, the *systolic pressure,* normally about 120 millimeters of mercury (mm Hg). During the next half second, the heart relaxes, referred to as *diastole,* and as blood drains out of the large arteries into the smaller branches, the pressure falls to its lowest level, the *diastolic pressure,* normally about 80 mm Hg. Thus, the normal blood pressure in the aorta and large arteries is about 120 over 80, or 120/80 mm Hg. This is the pressure usually measured at the elbow over the large artery that supplies blood to the arm.

The heart contains two receiving chambers (atria) and two pumping chambers (ventricles), which are connected through a system of valves (Figure 5). The right atrium and ventricle are separated by a thick band of muscle from the left atrium and ventricle so that the oxygen-depleted blood returning to the right side of the heart from the body does not mix with the oxygen-enriched blood returning to the left side of the heart from the lungs. The heart muscle or *myocardium* (from *myo,* meaning muscle, and *cardium,* meaning heart) performs a tremendous amount of work. Though it weighs less than a pound, it drives a little over two ounces of blood with each beat through some 60,000 miles of blood vessels to supply nourishment to the trillions of cells in the body. Beating 70 times a

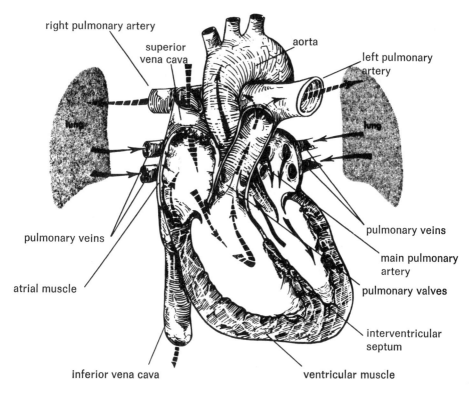

right pulmonary artery

superior
vena cava

aorta

left pulmonary
artery

lung

lung

pulmonary veins

atrial muscle

pulmonary veins

main pulmonary
artery

pulmonary valves

interventricular
septum

inferior vena cava

ventricular muscle

Figure 5. A view of the human heart showing the direction of blood
flow by the arrows.

minute, over a 70-year lifetime, it pumps more than 2.5 billion
times to circulate more than 100 million gallons of blood.

The heart muscle must constantly be supplied with fresh
blood through its own system of arteries, capillaries, and veins.
The arteries supplying the myocardium are called the *coronary*
arteries (from the Latin word for "crown") because they lie
over the surface of the heart like an upside-down crown.

The heartbeat is controlled by electrical impulses originating

15

in a "node" or pacemaker in the wall of the right atrium. These electrical impulses traverse the heart muscle and may be recorded from the surface of the chest by an electrocardiogram (ECG).

The large arteries branching from the aorta must constantly withstand a high head of pressure and repeatedly stretch back and forth like a rubber band with each heartbeat—expanding to hold the blood squeezed out of the heart during the period of contraction (systole), tightening to push the blood on through the circulation into the tissues during the period of relaxation (diastole). To perform their work, the walls of these larger arteries must contain considerable elastic tissue and muscle.

THE NATURE OF CARDIOVASCULAR DISEASE

A system as intricate and hardworking as the heart and circulation is susceptible to various damages and dysfunctions. Some of these are present at birth (congenital), arising from defects in the development of the system. Some arise from infections attacking the heart valves or muscle—rheumatic fever, bacterial endocarditis, myocarditis, and so forth. Other dysfunctions reflect damage to the heart muscle (cardiomyopathy) from various toxins, the most common being alcohol, weakening the power of the pump mechanism and leading to heart failure.

But our concern is the most common and serious form of cardiovascular disease, caused by the development of "rust" in the walls of the arteries throughout the body and primarily in the coronary arteries supplying the heart muscle (myocardium) itself. This "rust" is composed of fat and cholesterol which deposit in the walls of the arteries in the form of plaques, called *atheromas*. As the fatty atheroma embeds within the arterial walls, the vessels lose some of their elasticity and strength, becoming progressively thicker and more rigid. This hardening of the arterial wall by atheroma is re-

16

ferred to as *sclerosis* and the entire process is called *atherosclerosis,* or hardening of the arteries (Figure 6). Atherosclerosis is responsible for most of the heart attacks, strokes, and other vascular catastrophes that, in turn, kill and maim more people than any other pathological process afflicting mankind.

Some atherosclerosis is an expected accompaniment of the wear and tear of normal life. But the process can be accelerated by various factors that we will consider in more detail. First, let us see the consequences of atherosclerosis—hardening of the arteries or rust in the pipes.

As in any set of pipes carrying fluid, problems may occur when rust begins to accumulate: the flow of fluid may be slowed or stopped or the wall may become so weak that it ruptures. In our bodies, these processes cause different problems depending upon how extensive they are, how suddenly they develop, and where they occur.

Coronary Artery Disease

Atherosclerosis of the coronary arteries is responsible for most heart attacks. The process usually develops slowly, presumably beginning in childhood but only becoming manifest in late adult life. Atherosclerosis advances over the decades but enough blood flows past the plaques to keep the heart muscle healthy and the person shows no symptoms—though the coronary arteries are diseased.

Then, suddenly, trouble appears: the plaque builds up enough to slow the flow of blood to the heart muscle supplied by that artery. If the heart muscle is only partially deprived of oxygen and other nutrients, it sets off pain, called *angina,* which is felt under the breastbone (sternum) or elsewhere in the upper body. This anginal pain often appears initially only when the heart is called upon to increase its work—during physical exertion, after an emotional upset, or following a heavy meal. As the process advances, the flow of blood may be inadequate even when the person is at rest. Such angina indi-

17

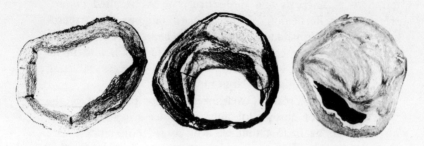

| Normal artery | Fatty deposits in vessel wall | Plugged artery with fatty deposits and clot |

Figure 6. A cross-section of human arteries, the left one normal, the middle with some fatty deposits (atheroma), the right with extensive atherosclerosis and a blood clot plugging the lumen.

cates more severe atherosclerosis and presages permanent damage to the heart muscle.

Either because an additional burden is placed on an already compromised circulation or because the artery becomes completely blocked, the heart muscle supplied by the artery, deprived of oxygen and other nutrients, cannot survive. The death of heart muscle is a heart attack or *myocardial infarction* (MI) (infarction means death of tissue because of inadequate blood supply). In the last few years, cardiologists have recognized that some angina and infarcts occur from temporary spasm of the arterial muscle (vasospasm), rather than from permanent obstruction. If the spasm persists, the end result is equally severe. The flow of blood may be obstructed by the development of a clot of blood (thrombus) over the surface of an atherosclerotic plaque. This surface is often jagged and irregular, providing a place where blood cells may accumulate and set off the process by which a clot forms. Within vessels supplying the heart, a *coronary thrombosis* may precipitate a heart attack.

18

The Consequences of a Heart Attack

Once a section of heart muscle dies, one of a number of events transpires:

- In a surprisingly large number of people, the event is passed over as "heartburn" or just another episode of anginal pain. Only when the heart is examined after death at a later time are old scars of prior infarcts identified. In most cases, the anginal pain persists or worsens and is accompanied by nausea, weakness, and sweating—enough to send the sufferer to the emergency room. There an electrocardiogram usually displays evidence of heart muscle damage and the diagnosis of an "acute MI" is confirmed. Admission to a Coronary Care Unit (CCU) is usual, to begin a two-to-six-week period of observation and rehabilitation. If the amount of heart muscle damage is marked, the necessary pumping function cannot be maintained and additional measures must be used to assist the circulation.

- In an unfortunate 20 to 30 percent of heart attack victims, death occurs suddenly, within minutes. This usually indicates an electrical disturbance in the heart rhythm, set off in the area of damaged muscle. The heart muscle quivers ineffectually, unable to contract and relax in the usual repetitive beat. The circulation ceases. Unless immediate cardiopulmonary resuscitation (CPR) is provided, death occurs within a few minutes because the brain cannot survive more than about four minutes without fresh blood.

  The saddest feature of these sudden deaths

is that many occur in hearts made irritable by
spasm without very extensive underlying damage to the heart muscle. If CPR is provided
quickly, survival may be possible.

· For most victims, the infarcted tissue gradually
forms a scar, but enough good heart tissue
remains to provide necessary pumping action.
However, the chances of repeated heart attacks are great.

Strokes or Cerebral Vascular Disease

A similar process of progressive atherosclerosis frequently
occurs in the arteries that supply the brain, the *cerebral* vessels.
The manifestation of insufficient blood flow to the brain tissue, however, is not pain. Rather, brain function is lost. If the
event is only temporary—a transient ischemic attack or TIA
(ischemia refers to decreased blood supply)—a brief spell of
numbness, muscle weakness, or partial blindness may be noted.
If it's more persistent, the affected brain tissue is permanently
damaged, resulting in a *stroke* or cerebral vascular accident
(CVA). The loss of sensation, muscle function, speech, or
other brain function persists, though other brain areas may
take over and functions slowly return.

In the cerebral circulation, weak spots within the smaller
arteries may suddenly rupture, the escape of blood under high
pressure rapidly damaging the rather soft, gelatinous brain
tissue. These *cerebral hemorrhages* are particularly common
in those who have a history of elevated blood pressure. Such
hemorrhages may be heralded by a severe headache and may
quickly lead to coma and death.

Other Vascular Diseases

Atherosclerotic narrowing and rupture may occur throughout
the arterial system. Certain vessels are particularly susceptible
in special circumstances: the kidney vessels in blacks with

hypertension, the arteries in the legs of diabetics. Perhaps the most common area is within the major artery coming out of the heart, the aorta. Some aortic atherosclerosis is usual in those over age 50, but in some the vessel wall may weaken and bulge, forming an *aneurysm*. In others, a tear develops which may either dissect a false channel down the vessel or rupture through the wall.

Though these other cardiovascular events have serious consequences, they are relatively infrequent, compared to heart attacks and strokes. Therefore, our attention will remain focused on these two, and primarily on heart attacks. Recall their frequency in the United States each year: over 1.2 million heart attacks, with nearly 650,000 deaths from coronary heart disease, over 150,000 in people under age 65; over 400,000 strokes, with 175,000 deaths, at least 25,000 in people younger than age 65.

THE CAUSES OF CARDIOVASCULAR DISEASE

We now leave an area of great certainty—there's little doubt about death rates and the causes of death—to one of inferences, associations, and likelihoods. We do not know for certain what causes most cardiovascular disease, in particular the atherosclerotic coronary artery disease responsible for most heart attacks. But we have some very strong circumstantial evidence pointing to a number of factors that increase the risk of developing coronary disease. These are called risk factors or disease predictors.

Just as poor sanitation, overcrowding, poverty, and malnutrition unquestionably contributed to the development and spread of tuberculosis in the nineteenth century, so high blood pressure, cigarette smoking, and high cholesterol contribute to the development of atherosclerosis and, in turn, cardiovascular disease today. The specific cause of tuberculosis is a microorganism, the Mycobacterium tuberculosis. Even before the tubercle bacillus was identified and long before specific antibiotic treatment was available, improvements in sanitation and living conditions resulted in a marked decrease in the prevalence of that dread disease.

So it is with atherosclerosis. The specific cause remains unknown and we cannot with any certainty cure it. But if we reduce the prevalence and severity of the various risk factors for atherosclerosis, we can just as surely control the current epidemic of cardiovascular disease.

Identifying the Risk Factors

A number of large-scale, long-term epidemiological studies have identified certain characteristics that are associated with the development of cardiovascular disease. Perhaps the most widely known of these is the Framingham Study, begun in 1948 in Framingham, Massachusetts, in which 5,127 people between the ages of 30 and 60 have been intensively tested every two years. From the hundreds of facts known about the participants—their habits, histories, physical characteristics, and the results of laboratory tests—it has been possible to relate the development of various diseases over the ensuing 30 years to features that were present initially or which developed subsequently.

Typically, those who developed a heart attack or stroke were more likely to smoke cigarettes and to have high blood pressure and a high blood cholesterol—the three major risk factors (see Table 1). In addition, more of them were overweight, physically inactive, under greater emotional stress, and diabetic (all rated as minor risk factors).

Studies such as the Framingham Study do not—cannot—prove a direct cause and effect relation. That can only be done by taking a large number of people without a given risk factor, such as cigarette smoking, who are free of cardiovascular disease, and having them take on the risk factor—smoke regularly for a long period of time—while being carefully monitored for the development of disease. These people would be continuously compared to another large group of people similar in every way except that they do not smoke.

Table 1: The Known Risk Factors for Cardiovascular Disease	
Major	**Minor**
Cigarette smoking	Obesity
Hypercholesterolemia	Physical inactivity
Hypertension	Diabetes and glucose intolerance
	Stress and personality type
	Excessive alcohol intake
	Estrogen intake

Such human experimentation is well nigh impossible. Consider that the nonsmokers might still be exposed to enough noxious substances from other people's smoke to develop some of the trouble that is caused by cigarettes. It would not be feasible to control the large number of people needed for such a definitive study.

Therefore, we depend upon studies such as Framingham to point to associations. For a factor to be accepted as a likely cause of a disease—as with cigarette smoking and heart disease—a number of "proofs" must be evident:

- The risk factor must be shown to have been present before the disease develops.
- There must be a strong association which increases progressively with greater exposure to the risk.
- The association must be consistently observed in multiple, different populations.
- The association must be independent of other risk factors (smokers could get heart disease because they had higher blood pressure).
- The association must be plausible, in keeping with what is known about the cause of the disease (as we shall see, smoking involves a number of things that can damage the heart).

23

- The association is supported by experiments in animals.
- Removal of the risk where possible is shown to decrease the occurrence of the disease.

In the chapters that follow, each of the important risk factors will be examined with the aim of showing how they cause trouble, and, more important, how you can avoid or remove them from your "risk profile."

Other Ways to Look at Risk Factors

Let us look further at the classification of the risk factors for cardiovascular disease shown in Table 1. High blood pressure, cigarette smoking, and high blood cholesterol are called the "major" risks because:

1. They are present in a significant proportion of the population.
2. If present, they are more likely than other factors to be associated with the disease.
3. Among those who develop the disease, they are the risks most frequently noted.

On the other hand, a risk listed as "minor" may be quite important for some people. If you are diabetic, for example, your risk of developing cardiovascular disease is quite high. But only about 2 percent of the entire population are diabetic. Therefore, for the other 98 percent, diabetes is a "minor" risk.

Dr. William Kannel, one of the primary directors of the Framingham Study, has proposed another classification of risk factors, based primarily upon how they arise (Table 2). Neither his list nor Table 1 is meant to include every possibility. In a 1981 survey of all medical publications, Drs. Paul N. Hopkins and Roger R. Williams found a total of 246 possible risk factors for coronary artery disease. Nonetheless, Tables 1 and 2 identify the more important risks, and they will be the ones considered in the following chapters.

THE PUZZLE OF HEART DISEASE

Table 2: Classification of Risk Factors for Cardiovascular Disease*

Personal Attributes That Promote Atherosclerosis
High blood pressure
High blood cholesterol
Diabetes
Gout

Living Habits
Cigarette smoking
High intake of saturated fats
High intake of sodium
Obesity
Physical inactivity
Excessive alcohol intake
Use of oral contraceptives
Psychosocial influences
Environmental factors: water hardness, trace metals, climate, air pollution

Personal Susceptibility to Develop Atherosclerosis
Racial and ethnic patterns
Family history
Post-menopausal state
Male sex
Older age

Preclinical Signs of Disease

* Dr. William Kannel, personal communication.

Before proceeding to the individual risk factors, a few comments about the genetic connection seem appropriate. If you inherit "bad" genes which predispose you to a disease, you may consider your fate to be predetermined and impossible to change.

In fact, virtually every inherited condition that predisposes to cardiovascular disease—and that includes at least high

25

blood pressure, high cholesterol, and diabetes—needs a certain environment in which to develop and cause trouble. Thus, if someone in your family has hypertension, you are more likely to develop high blood pressure, but that likelihood is even more enhanced if you eat lots of sodium, become overweight, and live under high levels of stress. Your chances of developing hypertension will be reduced if you avoid these environmental provocations.

So rather than taking a defeatist attitude, consider the presence of cardiovascular disease in your family as a helpful warning signal. Even if you can't identify a specific inherited condition, the fact that a close family member died or suffered from cardiovascular disease should be a warning. Careful attention to your health and living habits will help you to avoid cardiovascular disease.

Single versus Multiple Causes

The large number of risk factors that exist does bring up an important—and frustrating—aspect of the problem of cardiovascular disease. We have all become enamored of the idea of the "Magic Bullet"—the theory that every disease has a specific cause and that, therefore, a specific cure can be pinpointed. This idea arose with the remarkable discoveries of Pasteur and Ehrlich and other nineteenth- and early twentieth-century "microbe hunters," who were able to find the specific causes and cures for a number of infectious diseases.

Unfortunately, most noninfectious diseases don't follow the specific cause-specific cure model. Perhaps as we uncover more about the very beginnings of heart disease and cancer, "magic bullets" will be found. But our present information indicates that these diseases arise from the interactions of multiple factors, some inherited, most acquired from the environment in which we live.

One further disclaimer about "magic bullets": don't be misled into thinking that it doesn't matter if you develop heart disease—that before long, we'll be able to replace the old one with a brand new model. Nothing could be farther from the truth as we know it at present. Even if all of the problems of rejection, infection, and so on could be solved and the cost of over $100,000 paid for, there is absolutely no way for any but a handful of people to have a heart transplant, for there are so few normal, healthy hearts available. And what would happen to the transplant if we exposed it to all of the bad habits responsible for the trouble with the original heart?

Each risk factor increases the likelihood of developing cardiovascular disease and, in general, the more of each, the greater the likelihood. You may have very high levels of one or another, making you a very high risk. But more likely, you've got just a small amount of a number of risks—a slightly elevated blood pressure, a few extra pounds of weight, an occasional binge of booze. In small degrees, none of these risk factors is associated with a great deal of potential trouble. But unfortunately, they interact and, in a sense, multiply each other's impact. The figures in Table 3 indicate the relative degree of risk of having a heart attack, using age, blood cholesterol, systolic blood pressure, and number of cigarettes smoked each day. To derive the overall risk, you must *multiply* all the factors together. Take a 48-year-old person with a cholesterol of 290, a systolic blood pressure of 165, who smokes 20 cigarettes a day:

$$1.36 \times 2.20 \times 2.80 \times 2.40 = 20.2$$

1.36	×	2.20	×	2.80	×	2.40	=	20.2
(risk for age)		(risk for cholesterol)		(risk for blood pressure)		(risk for smoking)		(relative risk)

Thus, this person would have a 20.2 times greater risk of having a heart attack than a 40-year-old nonsmoker with normal cholesterol and blood pressure.

To reduce the risk of a heart attack, most of us must try to correct and change a number of different habits and traits. The good news in all of this is that the degree of change in life-style that is needed for most of us should not be that difficult to achieve.

Table 3: Relative Risk Factors for Coronary Heart Disease (CHD) with Predictive Values for U.S. Populations*

Age (Years)	Risk of CHD	Cholesterol (mg/100 ml)	Risk of CHD	Systolic Blood Pressure (mm Hg)	Risk of CHD	Smoking (cigarettes/day)	Risk of CHD
40–44	1.00	<180	0.74	<115	0.73	None	1.00
45–49	1.36	to 229	1.00	to 129	1.00	<5	1.25
50–54	1.84	to 289	1.61	to 159	1.70	to 9	1.56
55–59	2.40	to 299	2.20	to 169	2.80	to 19	1.95
≧60	2.50	≧300	3.00	≧170	5.00	to 29	2.40
						≧30	3.00

* From T. Khosla *et al.*, "Who is at Risk of a Coronary?" *British Medical Journal*, February 5, 1977, p. 342.

HOW TO
CALCULATE YOUR RISK STATUS

Table 3 can be used to approximate your own current risk status relative to the general U.S. population. It's as good as any and better than most of the tables, lists, tests, and games that have been used to determine relative risk. Another self-scoring test that includes an estimate of weight, physical activity, and stress level is shown in Table 4. Remember that these are only approximations and cannot take all possible factors into account. Most are based on the observations made in the Framingham Study and they can be projected for only a six- to eight-year period. The risk profile provides you with a good idea of your potential for developing cardiovascular disease. The higher your relative risk, the more diligent you'll need to be to reduce your current risk factors.

But even if you score low in these tests, don't assume you're a low risk. We in the United States have one of the world's highest rates of cardiovascular disease. Should we regard the "average" risk for Americans as our goal? Perhaps we can't get down to the level of the Japanese, whose rate of death from heart disease is less than one-sixth of ours. But why shouldn't we do as well as the French, or the Italians, or any of the other groups whose rate is half of ours?

SOCIETY AND THE INDIVIDUAL

Thus far the emphasis has been on each individual's risks and the need to take whatever action is necessary to remove them. For the relatively small proportion of the population at high risk—perhaps the top 5 percent—that course is essential. But remember that most of us have small amounts of many risks, and a great deal of cardiovascular disease will develop among people with relatively small individual risks. For the majority, we must take major action to reduce the overall risks as much as possible. For example:

- Smoking must be actively discouraged in every reasonable manner. Those who do take it up or

29

Table 4: A Self-Scoring Test for Cardiovascular Risk

Risk Factor	Score	
Smoking	0	Nonsmoker
	2	Fewer than 20 cigarettes a day
	4	20 cigarettes or more a day
Systolic blood pressure	0	Under 120
	2	120 to 140
	4	Over 140
Cholesterol level	0	Under 200
	2	200 to 250
	4	Over 250
Weight	0	Desirable
	2	10 to 20 percent over
	4	More than 20 percent over
Physical activity	0	Regular vigorous exercise
	2	Moderate exercise
	4	Sedentary
Stress and tension	0	Rarely tense or anxious
	2	Feel tense two or three times a day
	4	Extremely tense
Total risk	0–4	Low
	5–9	Below average
	10–14	Average
	15–20	High
	21–24	Very high

continue the habit obviously can't be forced to stop, but there's no reason to encourage cigarette smoking as is now being done.
· Sodium is added in excess amounts to virtually every processed food, and we have no way of

knowing how much is present. Here again, better to stop the harmful practice. But at the least, let it be made clear what is being added, so we can make our own choices.

· Infant feeding practices often promote the development of bad habits—the consumption of high saturated fat, high sodium, and excess calories—that continue into adult life. There should be a widespread program of education to make parents aware of these problems.

The list could go on and on. As a society, we must take these and other reasonable and prudent steps to stop the epidemic of cardiovascular disease. Not only will this approach reduce the likelihood that the small group at high-risk will be protected, but, more important, it will help the majority of us who are at relatively smaller risk.

The British epidemiologist Geoffrey Rose has put the "strategy of prevention" into an interesting perspective. Taking the control of hypertension as a model, he has compared the potential benefits from our current "high-risk" strategy of detecting and treating those who already have high blood pressure to those of a total community strategy, in which a modest reduction in sodium intake would lower overall blood pressure by two or three millimeters of mercury. He concludes that "all of the life saving benefits achieved by current antihypertensive treatment might be equalled by a downward shift of the whole blood pressure distribution in the population by a mere 2–3 mm Hg. The benefits from a mass approach in which everybody receives a small benefit may be unexpectedly large."[1]

So, as we consider the risk factors in the following chapters, let us keep the larger picture in focus. All of us, low and high risk, need to encourage good health habits for ourselves, our families, and our entire society.

31

THREE

Smoking

Smoking is perhaps the single most preventable cause of cardio-vascular disease. Though the fact that cigarette smokers tend to die earlier than nonsmokers was first reported by Dr. Raymond Pearl in 1938, it wasn't until 1964 that the dangers of smoking were clearly and conclusively documented. Since then, from 15 to 30 million Americans have quit, but their places have been largely taken by teenagers who have continued to take up the habit.

Most of this chapter will relate to cigarette smoking. Though pipes, cigars, snuff, and chewing tobacco may also present problems, they tend to be much less serious. However, if those who switch from cigarettes to cigars and pipes continue to inhale, they will most likely suffer the same consequences. Danish cheroot smokers have been found to have an even higher risk of heart attacks than cigarette smokers.

THE SCOPE OF THE PROBLEM

Some 53 million Americans smoke, even though two-thirds say they would like to quit. Each year, about 325,000 Americans die prematurely as a direct consequence of their smoking. Of these deaths about 75,000 are due to cancer of the lung. Less well recognized by most people is the fact that the largest number of smoking-related deaths are cardiovascular in nature.

The more you smoke, the more trouble you'll have. The rate of heart attack for white males aged 30 to 59 almost triples between those who are nonsmokers and those who smoke more than one pack per day.

Cigarette smoke contains over 4,000 components, so it is not certain which of them are responsible for the production of cardiovascular disease. Most likely, it's a combination of the effects of nicotine and carbon monoxide.

Nicotine is a direct stimulant to the heart muscle, causing a rise in heart rate and blood pressure even in an addicted smoker. In addition, nicotine sets off the release of the hormone adrenaline from the adrenal gland, which whips the heart to even greater action. The stimulated heart needs more oxygen. If the coronary arteries are partially blocked by buildup of atherosclerotic plaque, smoking may bring on angina. Further, nicotine may set up disturbances in the rhythm of the heartbeat, and in the long term it may actually lead to the development of more atherosclerosis.

Interestingly, pipe smokers, who may absorb as much nicotine as do cigarette smokers, don't have more coronary disease than nonsmokers, so it is likely that other components of cigarette smoke are working in concert with the nicotine.

Carbon monoxide, another toxic material in cigarette smoke, may be the major factor in causing cardiovascular disease. The incomplete combustion of organic materials in tobacco gives rise to carbon monoxide (CO), which is inhaled and rapidly absorbed into the blood. Carbon monoxide attaches itself firmly to the hemoglobin in red blood cells, stripping off the oxygen which the hemoglobin normally carries to the various tissues. The blood of cigarette smokers has been found to contain, on the average, 20 percent less oxygen. As a result, heart muscle and other tissues may not receive enough oxygen for normal function.

In people who have underlying coronary disease, the small amounts of carbon monoxide inhaled from other people's smoke in poorly ventilated rooms or while driving in heavy traffic may set off angina.

Whatever elements are responsible, and nicotine and carbon monoxide are only two of the likely candidates, smokers have more atherosclerosis in their coronary blood vessels, experience more frequent heart attacks, and have a greater chance of dying suddenly after a heart attack. Furthermore, almost immediately after stopping smoking, the incidence of heart attacks and sudden death goes down. Other ill effects take longer to dissipate, however, and some, such as the scarring of lung tissue that causes emphysema, may never go away.

Other vascular problems, particularly peripheral vascular disease, are also more common in smokers than nonsmokers. The risk for stroke is about 1.5 times greater. Most of the clinical events occur in those with underlying atherosclerosis. Therefore, those who have hypertension, high blood cholesterol, or diabetes are more likely to suffer. A particularly strong link to heart attacks has been noted in women over age 35 who smoke and take oral contraceptives.

WHY YOU SMOKE

Young people often start smoking in response to pressure from their peers to appear more mature. They get considerable encouragement from the example of their smoking parents and from the media. As many as one in four 17 year olds is a regular smoker even though most are aware of the long-term dangers of smoking.

Because they perceive most of the hazards of smoking—such as cancer and emphysema—as long-term problems, many believe it is all right to smoke for a while and then to quit before troubles develop. But once they've smoked regularly most are addicted and can't easily shake the habit.

Cigarettes are probably more addictive than alcohol or barbiturates. Few smokers can use tobacco only occasionally, whereas most people who drink alcohol or take sleeping pills can do without them for long periods. Moreover, dependence on alcohol or drugs usually develops on a background of psychological distress or social upheaval, while addiction to tobacco occurs without such emotional factors.

For whatever reason smoking is taken up, it is the nicotine that appears to cause the addiction. With each puff of smoke, a small quantity of nicotine, 50 to 150 micrograms, is absorbed through the lining of the mouth and lungs: a total of one to two milligrams per cigarette. Nicotine is a very potent drug with multiple actions within the brain. Just which of these actions is responsible for addiction is unknown but, before long, a nicotine boost is needed every 20 to 30 minutes during waking hours to prevent the development of withdrawal symptoms.

The Self-Help Stop Smoking Program of the American Cancer Society has devised a "Smoker's Self-Awareness Profile" to help people ascertain why they continue to smoke, because an awareness of the nature and extent of the habit is an important part of the behavioral-modification approach toward breaking it. The first test in the profile has been reprinted here, along with the interpretations. The Smoker's Self-Awareness Profile was developed from material provided by the National Clearinghouse for Smoking and Health of the Bureau of Health Education, Center for Disease Control, in Atlanta.

Smoker's Self-Awareness Profile

Test 1—Why Do You Smoke?

Here are some statements made by people to describe what they get out of smoking cigarettes. How *often* do you feel this way when smoking them? Circle one number for each statement.

Important: Answer every question.

	Always	Frequently	Occasionally	Seldom	Never
A. I smoke cigarettes in order to keep myself from slowing down.	5	4	3	2	1

	Always	Fre-quently	Occa-sionally	Seldom	Never
B. Handling a cigarette is part of the enjoyment of smoking it.	5	4	3	2	1
C. Smoking cigarettes is pleasant and relaxing.	5	4	3	2	1
D. I light up a cigarette when I feel angry about something.	5	4	3	2	1
E. When I have run out of cigarettes I find it almost unbearable until I can get them.	5	4	3	2	1
F. I smoke cigarettes automatically without even being aware of it.	5	4	3	2	1
G. I smoke cigarettes to stimulate me, to perk myself up.	5	4	3	2	1
H. Part of the enjoyment of smoking a cigarette comes from the steps I take to light up.	5	4	3	2	1
I. I find cigarettes pleasurable.	5	4	3	2	1

	Always	Fre-quently	Occa-sionally	Seldom	Never
J. When I feel uncomfortable or upset about something, I light up a cigarette.	5	4	3	2	1
K. I am very much aware of the fact when I am not smoking a cigarette.	5	4	3	2	1
L. I light up a cigarette without realizing I still have one burning in the ashtray.	5	4	3	2	1
M. I smoke cigarettes to give me a "lift."	5	4	3	2	1
N. When I smoke a cigarette, part of the enjoyment is watching the smoke as I ex-hale it.	5	4	3	2	1
O. I want a cigarette most when I am comfortable and relaxed.	5	4	3	2	1
P. When I feel "blue" or want to take my mind off cares and worries, I smoke cigarettes.	5	4	3	2	1

	Always	Fre-quently	Occa-sionally	Seldom	Never
Q. I get a real gnaw-ing hunger for a cigarette when I haven't smoked for a while.	5	4	3	2	1
R. I've found a cigarette in my mouth and didn't remember putting it there.	5	4	3	2	1

How to Score:

1. Enter the numbers you have circled to the Test 1 questions in the spaces below, putting the number you have circled to Question A over line A, to Question B over line B, etc.
2. Total the 3 scores on each line to get your totals. For example, the sum of your scores over lines A, G, and M gives you your score on *Stimulation*—lines B, H, and N give the score on *Handling*, etc.

				Totals
____ A	+ ____ G	+ ____ M	=	_____ **Stimulation**
____ B	+ ____ H	+ ____ N	=	_____ **Handling**
____ C	+ ____ I	+ ____ O	=	_____ **Pleasurable Relaxation**
____ D	+ ____ J	+ ____ P	=	_____ **Crutch: Tension Reduction**
____ E	+ ____ K	+ ____ Q	=	_____ **Craving: Psychological Addiction**

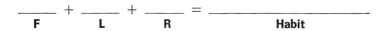

_____	+ _____	+ _____	=	_____
F	**L**	**R**		**Habit**

Scores can vary from 3 to 15. Any score 11 and above is high; any score 7 and below is low.

What Your Scores on Test 1 Tell About Why You Smoke

What kind of smoker are you? What do you get out of smoking? What does it do for you? This test is designed to provide you with a score on each of 6 factors which describe many people's smoking. Your smoking may be well characterized by only one of these factors, or by a combination of factors.

A score of 11 or above on any factor indicates that this factor is an important source of satisfaction for you. The higher your score (15 is the highest), the more important a particular factor is in your smoking and the more useful the discussion of that factor can be in your attempt to quit.

1. Stimulation

If you score high or fairly high on this factor, it means that you are one of those smokers who are stimulated by the cigarette—you feel that it helps wake you up, organizes your energies, and keeps you going. If you try to give up smoking, you may want a safe substitute *(a brisk walk* or moderate exercise, for example), whenever you feel the urge to smoke.

2. Handling

Handling things can be satisfying, but there are many ways to keep your hands busy without lighting up or playing with a cigarette. Why not toy with a pen or pencil? Or try doodling. Or play with a coin, a piece of jewelry, or some other harmless object.

3. Accentuation of pleasure—pleasurable relaxation

It is not always easy to find out whether you use the cigarette to feel *good,* that is, get real, honest pleasure out of smoking (Factor 3) or keep from feeling so *bad* (Factor 4). About two-thirds of smokers score high or fairly high on *accentuation of*

39

pleasure, and about half of those also score as high or higher on *reduction of negative feelings*.

Those who do get real pleasure out of smoking often find that an honest consideration of the harmful effects of their habit is enough to help them quit.

4. Reduction of negative feelings, or "crutch"

Many smokers use the cigarette as a kind of crutch in moments of stress or discomfort, and on occasion it may work; the cigarette is sometimes used as a tranquilizer. But the heavy smoker, the person who tries to handle severe personal problems by smoking many times a day, is apt to discover that cigarettes do not help him deal with his problems effectively.

5. "Craving" or psychological addiction

Quitting smoking is difficult for the person who scores high on this factor—that of psychological addiction. For him, the craving for the next cigarette begins to build up the moment he puts one out.

Giving up cigarettes may be so difficult and cause so much discomfort that once he does quit, he will find it easy to resist the temptation to go back to smoking because he knows that some day he will have to go through the same agony again.

6. Habit

This kind of smoker is no longer getting much satisfaction from his cigarettes. He just lights them frequently without even realizing he is doing so. He may find it easy to quit and stay off if he can break the habit patterns he has built up. Cutting down gradually may be quite effective if there is a change in the way the cigarettes are smoked and the conditions under which they are smoked. The key to success is becoming *aware* of each cigarette you smoke. This can be done by asking yourself, "Do I really want this cigarette?" You may be surprised at how many you do not want.

HOW YOU CAN QUIT SMOKING

Because the hazards of smoking are obvious and because smoking is becoming more and more socially unacceptable, you most likely want to quit. For most habituated smokers, quitting is difficult and there are literally hundreds of Stop-Smoking programs. Most help about two-thirds of the people who take them to quit, but, after a year, at least half have re-started. Nonetheless anybody—even the most hard-core, four-pack-a-day, 40-year smoker—can quit. What is essential is your unequivocal commitment to quitting. All of the various programs provide help to make it easier and to strengthen your willpower. But if you really aren't ready, it's unlikely that anything will work permanently. It's just too easy to start up again. Don't give up the fight, though: each day without a cigarette is a better day for your health.

A Safer Cigarette?

Probably you have switched from nonfiltered, high-nicotine cigarettes—there aren't too many of the old Camels' smokers still around—to a filtered, low-nicotine cigarette. With the increasing public awareness of the health consequences of smoking, cigarette manufacturers quickly responded by providing what everyone assumed to be a "safer cigarette."

Don't be fooled. The lower tar content of Carltons, Nows, and so on does offer you some protection against lung cancer. But they do not protect you from the major danger of heart disease. Remember what you are addicted to—nicotine—and what is most likely the major source of trouble in cigarettes—carbon monoxide. Now consider what happens when you switch from high-tar, high-nicotine Camels to low-tar, low-nicotine Carltons:

First, to get enough nicotine to satisfy your addiction, you'll most likely smoke twice as many cigarettes, smoking each one farther down the cigarette, drawing each puff in deeper and inhaling farther into your lungs.

Second, the amount of carbon monoxide you inhale may be *increased*. Not only are you putting more smoke into your lungs, but the amount of CO in each puff may be higher because of the nonporous paper used on many filters which keeps room air out of the tobacco smoke you inhale.

Some believe the cigarette companies purposely have foisted

41

these weaker cigarettes on the public to increase their sales despite a shrinking number of smokers. Regardless, don't be fooled—there is no safe cigarette now and there will likely never be a safe cigarette. Proof of this has come from the Framingham study: smokers of filtered cigarettes have been shown to suffer *more* heart attacks than smokers of nonfiltered cigarettes. So, if you want to quit, great. But don't kid yourself in believing that you can continue to smoke and protect your heart.

Some Stop-Smoking Programs

1. Self-help: The American Cancer Society's "I Quit" kit provides a variety of aids and a seven-day program. Numerous books and guides have been printed. In England, some success has been reported with the use of nicotine chewing-gum, the idea being that if you get the nicotine "fix" you'll give up the cigarettes. Kicking the habit seems preferable.

   Though the cold-turkey approach may work as well, the do-it-yourself program that will be described on page 43 should help you.

2. Group programs: The Seventh Day Adventists sponsor a five-day plan with lectures and group meetings. Smoke Enders have eight weekly meetings with a highly structured program emphasizing behavior modification, positive conditioning, and periodic reunions, at a cost of around $400.

   Individual or group hypnosis has been helpful for some.

3. Adverse conditioning: The Schick Program involves rapid smoking, with inhalation every six seconds until symptoms such as nausea, dizziness, or blurred vision occur, with the purpose of setting up adverse conditioning which will block subsequent smoking.

A Self-Help Program Based on Behavior Modification

The following has been adopted from a variety of sources and is a safe, sensible program that may work for you:

Identify your problem

1. The Smoker's Self-Awareness Profile on page 35 should help show you why you smoke. Also try keeping a list of all the excuses you have used to continue smoking.
2. Keep a diary of your smoking habit for one week. On a piece of paper inside your pack of cigarettes, record the time, circumstance, and the way you feel when you light each cigarette.
3. Analyze your current habit. See how often you smoke without thinking about what you're doing and the relation between certain activities (such as talking on the phone) and lighting up.

Make the commitment to stop

1. Find a time when your life should be relatively free of stress, out-of-town trips, and so forth. You will need peace and quiet and some support from family and friends.
2. List all of the reasons you believe that you should quit. If you can't counter all of the excuses you've had to continue smoking, talk to someone who has successfully quit or seek professional help.
3. Make a written contract with yourself for what you believe you can do in the next two weeks—preferably, that will be to quit smoking. Think about including a reward for success (a luxury that you've long denied

yourself) and a penalty for failure (how about a significant donation to the university that is the hated football rival of your alma mater).

4. Tell someone you love that you are going to quit and ask for their support.

Start cutting down

1. Build up needed support:
   · start a regular daily exercise program
   · have low-calorie snacks available
   · get yourself involved in some pleasant activities (reading, volunteer work, racetrack handicapping)
   · get plenty of sleep
   · take more time and use some new (or forgotten) techniques in sexual relations
2. Intensify your awareness of your smoking:
   · empty all your ashtrays into a plastic sack each day and keep them lined up where you can see them (you can easily relate them to the inside of your lungs)
   · buy another brand, one pack at a time
   · keep recording the circumstances and the way you feel when you light each cigarette
3. Begin to taper off your smoking (this should probably take a week, though you may try a few days):
   · based upon your analysis of your own diary, cut out those cigarettes you've smoked without thinking about them or feeling a strong desire for them
   · keep your cigarettes in a place not immediately accessible, away from the phone, your desk, as examples
   · limit yourself to a cigarette every hour, preferably at set times when you do not

feel the urge to smoke. With each puff, imagine (or feel) the unpleasant sensations. Smoke each cigarette more rapidly than usual so that you feel some unpleasant sensations

4. Substitute nonsmoking activities:
   - use a positive-imaging technique (close your eyes and imagine a pleasant scene) or a relaxation technique such as transcendental meditation or simply breathing deeply before engaging in those activities that ordinarily provoke an urge to smoke
   - when the urge strikes, chew gum, eat a carrot, suck on a cinnamon stick, use an astringent mouthwash, or just take a deep breath
   - keep yourself busy with pleasant tasks
   - if nothing else works, take a walk

Quit smoking

1. Some have found that another week of a more limited schedule with only four or five cigarettes a day is useful. If you are feeling confident, you may prefer to quit after the tapering program.
2. When you quit, get rid of every cigarette and match in your surroundings.
3. Be prepared for some withdrawal symptoms: warn your family and friends that you'll probably be as irritable as a grizzly bear, don't try to do intricate work like balancing the checkbook, don't call up your in-laws.
4. When you're really feeling shaky, nervous, sweaty, and anxious, talk to your spouse or a friend who's already gone through withdrawal. Go to a long movie or a Wagnerian opera.

5. Start congratulating yourself. In a few days, the acute symptoms will disappear and you should actually begin to feel better—less morning cough, more awareness of tastes, better breath. Flaunt your success, but be on guard for those situations where smoking is "natural"—cocktail parties, morning coffee breaks, and so on.

6. Collect the money you would have spent each day on cigarettes and buy the reward you put into your contract.

7. Be prepared for temporary failure. Despite all of the best intentions, a business reverse, a fight with your spouse, or some other problem may wreck your plans. If you smoke a cigarette, try to limit it to one and stop again. But if that's not possible, it's probably best to smoke away for a week or more and start all over again when the time seems right. Don't deflate your ego unnecessarily. Some of the strongest people have quit ten times before achieving success. But keep saying to yourself: "I can quit."

   Many are able to quit for some months or years but start again. Even after years of being off cigarettes, many continue to feel the urge on occasion. So don't be surprised at the tenacity of your addiction. Remember that millions have been successful and think of the lasting benefits you will achieve by quitting.

8. Don't let yourself use the excuse that you must start back because you're gaining weight. It's true that most people gain a few pounds when they quit (smokers actually weigh about ten pounds less than nonsmokers, on the average). That may be from a combination of needing another form of oral gratification,

having a sharper sense of taste, and removing the calorie-burning effects of nicotine (which work through the hormone adrenaline). Keep on a low-calorie diet and exercise more. The extra pounds will come back off.

9. Offer your help to others who want to quit. Become a volunteer worker for the Cancer Society or Lung Association. Talk to your children about never, ever starting to smoke. Join ASH (Action on Smoking and Health, 2013 H Street NW, Washington, D.C. 20006).

The Benefits of Quitting

Not only will you begin to feel better but you'll most likely live longer. You will be able to exercise more and breathe more easily. Within two years, a decrease in the frequency of heart attacks was evident among men aged 45 to 64 in Framingham who quit smoking (Figure 7). The rate of heart attacks was cut by more than half. It is true that some increased mortality (particularly from cancer and lung disease) persists for even fifteen years in those who have quit, but most of the excess will be removed.

Better Never to Have Started

Obviously, all of us—and our children—would be better off if we could prevent the start of smoking. Dr. Richard Evans, in Houston, and others have shown that teenagers can be convinced not to start smoking if the approach is directed at their immediate experiences and is presented in an appropriate manner. Other teenagers who do not smoke explain how it's possible to withstand and repulse peer pressures. The immediate benefits of not smoking are emphasized: your boyfriend or girlfriend will want to kiss you more if you don't have bad breath, you'll be better at sports if you can breathe more easily.

Beyond these educational programs, a number of broader remedies should help:

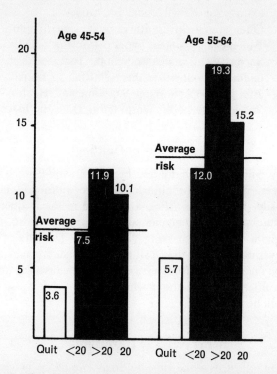

Figure 7. The average annual incidence of coronary events as related to smoking status among 45- to 64-year-old men in the Framingham, Massachusetts, study over an 18-year follow-up. The smoking habit refers to those who quit and those who smoke fewer than 20, 20, or more than 20 cigarettes a day. The number at the top of each bar is the number of cases of heart disease per 1,000 persons. (Source: Gordon, T. *et al., Lancet* 2 [1974]: 1345)

- Raise the cost by increasing taxes on cigarettes. They are almost $2.00 a pack in England. The cost of cigarettes has increased less than the Consumer Price Index over the past 20 years.
- Restrict advertising for cigarettes, particularly the seductive (use of athletes and fashion models) and misleading (sponsorship of sporting events) which induce children to start.
- Use advertising against smoking. The antismoking TV commercials shown in response to the equal-time fairness doctrine in 1968–1970 reduced cigarette consumption by 14 percent per year, causing the cigarette manufacturers to withdraw from all TV advertising.
- Increase the public's awareness of the dangers of smoking and parents' awareness of their role in subtly convincing their children to start smoking.
- Make it more difficult for children to buy cigarettes, enforcing restrictions as with the sale of alcohol.
- Ensure the rights of nonsmokers to clean air by prohibiting smoking in all public places.
- Stop government support of the tobacco farmers.

There is hope for the antismoking campaign. The steady increase in teenage smoking noted during the 1960s and early '70s appears to have peaked and actually receded. More and more adults have quit: it's almost impossible to find a smoker at most medical meetings; some airlines and hotels have a no-smoking policy. So as social demands and economic factors continue to strengthen the pro-health forces, we may find that we will be smoking less and living better and longer. Thank you for not smoking.

FOUR

Hypertension

The second of the major risk factors for cardiovascular disease is as common as cigarette smoking but much less obvious. Most who have hypertension—the medical term for high blood pressure—are without symptoms. Only if your blood pressure is taken will you know for sure. Even your friends can't tell you, unless they have a sphygmomanometer (blood pressure recorder).

THE NATURE OF HYPERTENSION

As described in chapter 2, the pressure within your heart and major arteries is normally around 120 (systolic)/over 80 (diastolic) millimeters of mercury (mm Hg). The level of blood pressure is lower during childhood, reaches adult levels at about age 16, and tends to remain fairly stable throughout the 20's and 30's. However, for the population at large, both the diastolic and, to an even greater degree, the systolic pressures tend to rise as we grow older—an increase that tends to be higher in blacks than in whites.

Though the average blood pressure rises, these averages cover an entire spectrum of readings, some of which remain quite low, others of which go up a bit, and still others rise markedly. Certain levels of blood pressure are labeled as "high" and the diagnosis of hypertension is affixed. For most adults, that level is anything above 140 systolic over 90 diastolic.

This criterion hasn't just been picked out of the air. It is based upon large-scale epidemiological studies such as Framingham that have shown that significantly more cardiovascular disease will appear among those whose pressures rise above 140 over 90.

Women seem not to suffer quite as much as men at any given level of blood pressure. However, more women end up with hypertension, so the relative risks tend to be equalized. Overall, almost 20 percent of the adult U.S. population have a blood pressure above 140/90, the number rising—as does the average blood pressure—with each increment of age.

Your pressure may have been recorded as normal on one occasion and high at another. Actually, your blood pressure is constantly changing, from minute to minute, as much as 20 to 30 mm Hg (or, as some prefer, "points"). When you sleep it may go down by 40 mm Hg, when you strain at stool it may go up by 60 mm Hg.

Even while you are seemingly relaxed, your pressure may bounce around considerably. Therefore, most physicians prefer to take three readings during an exam and take the average of these as the "true" reading. In the past few years, more and more people have been taking their own readings with home blood pressure kits. In order to know what the usual pressure is, three sets of readings at different times should be recorded.

Many readings need to be taken to ensure that a person is really hypertensive. The division between "high" and "normal" at 140/90 is somewhat arbitrary, since every millimeter of rise is associated with some increase in cardiovascular trouble. We've taken the 140/90 value as the dividing line because that's when a significant amount of trouble begins to show up, but that number really should be the average of a series of readings. Unless the readings are definitely dangerous (like

210/130), there's really no hurry to make the diagnosis. Often the first readings tend to be considerably higher, probably because the patient is tense.

Though it's a good idea to confirm those first readings, they shouldn't be disregarded even if all the subsequent ones are lower. At the least, such occasional high readings indicate that persistent high readings may develop. They should be taken as warning signals to continue watching the blood pressure and do what can be done to prevent a progressive rise.

THE CAUSES OF HYPERTENSION

Remember that the normal blood pressure reflects the force of the pumping action of the heart, squeezing blood into the large muscular arteries. The pressure within these arteries could increase by one of three processes:

1. The heart could pump harder and faster.
2. The amount of blood could increase, over-filling the circulation.
3. The capacity of the arteries could be decreased.

Each of these processes may be involved in the most common form of the disease, present in more than nine of ten persons with hypertension. Since a specific cause is not known, this form is called "primary," "idiopathic," or "essential," the latter term reflecting an old, mistaken notion that higher pressures might be needed to keep blood flowing through arteries narrowed with aging. The trigger that sets off the process is unknown, but the most plausible theory is that it starts by the slow retention by the kidneys of a small quantity of the large amount of sodium we eat daily. Presumably, the defect in kidney function is hereditary, since this form of hypertension tends to occur twice as often in children of hypertensive parents. Over many years, the buildup of sodium (and water) overfills the circulation and causes the pressure to rise. In an attempt to protect themselves from the heightened pressure, arteries become thicker. This, in turn, limits their capacity and further raises the pressure.

The Hidden Sodium in Our Foods

Theorizing that the cause of hypertension involves the slow retention of sodium, it follows that if little sodium is eaten (usually as table salt or sodium chloride) the blood pressure may not rise, even if the kidney defect is present. The frequency of hypertension is decidedly lower in certain primitive groups of people, scattered around the world, who do not eat the excessive amounts of sodium that we, the more civilized, have learned to love.

You are probably now eating about 10 to 15 grams (⅓ to ½ an ounce) of sodium chloride a day, approximately two to three flat teaspoonfuls. Most of this is present in the processed (frozen, canned, precooked) foods which comprise the mainstay of our diet. Why do these processed foods contain so much sodium? The most frequently given explanation is that it serves as a preservative. That may have been true before modern refrigeration and airtight packaging became available, but is no longer the case. It's there now because we like it and food processors, knowing what tastes we like, add the salt. In fact, until a few years ago, they even added large amounts of sodium to baby foods—not for any possible babies' needs but for the mothers' taste. They knew that mothers often tasted their baby's foods before feeding it to their infants. Infants, born without a need or desire for salt, soon developed a preference for it and thereafter grew into the salt-gobbling adults that you and I now are. In recent years, after the potential harm of this extra sodium was recognized, it has been left out, so perhaps the next generation will have less preference for sodium—and, one hopes, less hypertension.

The amount of sodium added to almost every processed food these days (mostly in the form of benzoate, glutamate, or other derivatives) is too little to serve as an adequate preservative. Unfortunately, you are very likely unaware of how much salt is in the foods you eat (see Table 5, "Sodium Content of

Table 5: Sodium Content of Some Processed Foods

	Amount	Sodium (mgs)
Tomato catsup (Heinz)	1 tbsp.	182
Frankfurter, beef (Oscar Mayer)	1	425
Bologna (Oscar Mayer)	2 slices	450
Tomato juice (Del Monte)	1 cup	640
Cinnamon rolls (Pillsbury)	1	630
Chicken noodle soup (Campbell's)	10 oz.	1050
Frozen turkey dinner (Swanson)	1	1735
Pickle, dill	1 large	1928

Some Processed Foods"). Would you believe there's more sodium in corn flakes than Fritos? What we need is the labeling of the sodium content of every processed food but, as of early 1982, only about 15 percent of processed foods were so labeled. As an alternative you can choose fresh, nonprocessed foods, which invariably have less sodium (see Table 6). As long as you don't overuse your saltshaker, your intake of salt will certainly diminish. But there's another problem: virtually every fast food—the source of more than one-third of the meals we consume—has lots of sodium. One order of three pieces of Kentucky Fried Chicken, mashed potatoes, and cole slaw has over 5 grams of salt or 2.3 grams of sodium—as much as we should consume in an entire day.

The evidence incriminating our current excessive sodium intake as the cause of hypertension is only circumstantial but it is impressive:

- As noted, those people who eat little sodium (some less than a tenth of a gram—a few grains a day) have little or no hypertension.
- In general, the more sodium in the average diet, the more hypertension in the population.
- Decreasing the sodium in the diet or remov-

Table 6: Similar Foods Containing Low or High Levels of Sodium

Low	High
Shredded wheat (Nabisco), 1 mg/oz.	Corn flakes (General Mills), 305 mg/oz.
Green beans, fresh, 5 mg/cup	Green beans, canned (Del Monte), 925 mg/cup
Orange juice, 2 mg/cup	Tomato juice, 640 mg/cup
Turkey, roasted, 70 mg/3 oz.	Turkey dinner (Swanson), 1735 mg
Ground beef, 57 mg/3 oz.	Frankfurter, beef, 425 mg

ing some of the sodium (and water) from the body by using diuretic drugs will lower the blood pressure.

- Animals can be bred to have a predisposition for hypertension if they are given high sodium diets. Presumably humans also need the combination of heredity and high sodium intake.

Maybe the evidence doesn't prove the connection but it's strong enough to call for a general reduction of our sodium intake. Even though only some of us are adversely affected by salt intake, we currently have no way to identify these people beforehand, so the safest course would be for all of us to cut down. We're not looking for a rigidly reduced, no-salt diet, only a moderate restriction to about half of what we're now eating. This can be accomplished by cutting down on highly salted foods and removing the saltshaker from the kitchen and from the table. Not only can that be accomplished with relative ease, *it can cause no harm.* That's obviously vital, since we should do nothing that could hurt the nonsusceptible majority in order to protect even a large minority.

Even in hot, humid climates, we need very little sodium in our diets. When we first start exercising in such climates, our sweat contains a fair amount of sodium but in just a few days processes are set off which cause our body to retain every bit of needed sodium. As long as we're eating a reasonably normal diet, we're sure to get all the sodium that's needed, even during August preseason football practice in Texas.

Other Possible Factors

The preceding may be more than you cared to know about sodium, but we need to be greatly concerned about hypertension and the need to prevent the condition. There are at least two other factors that may be involved: obesity and psychological stress. People who are more than 20 percent above their "ideal" weight have about twice as much hypertension as those who are at or near their ideal weight. If they can reduce, their blood pressures usually fall. Some people who are chronically under high levels of stress develop hypertension and one or another relaxation technique may lower the blood pressure. Chronic stress may be partly responsible for the higher frequency of hypertension among blacks.

Obviously, since the specific cause of most hypertension is not known, we can't be sure of the roles of sodium, stress, or obesity. But at least we can try to reduce all three and thereby—without causing harm—we may be able to stop the development of hypertension.

THE CONSEQUENCES OF HYPERTENSION

You may be wondering, why be concerned over preventing hypertension? Quite simply, because it is "the silent killer." The term is pertinent because it is usually both silent (until it's too late) and because it is a major killer. The frequency of every form of cardiovascular disease—stroke, heart attacks, heart failure, and peripheral vascular disease—is increased in the presence of hypertension. Hypertension's relationship with

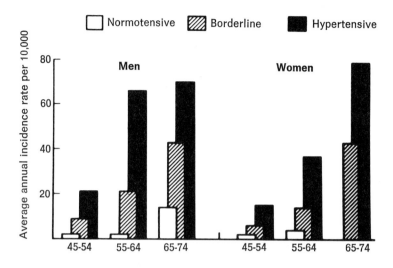

Figure 8. The average annual incidence rate for strokes (athero-thrombotic brain infarction) in men and women of varying ages in the Framingham, Massachusetts, study (18-year follow-up) classi-fied according to their level of blood pressure: normotensive = less than 140/90; borderline = 140/90 to 160/95; hypertensive = above 160/95. (Source: Kannel, W. B. *et al., Stroke* 7 [1976]: 327)

stroke is particularly striking (Figure 8). Let us consider how high blood pressure is transformed into these killer diseases.

High blood pressure causes trouble by acting as a purely mechanical stress upon the heart and blood vessels. The heart has to pump harder to squeeze blood against a higher head of pressure. The blood vessels are being flogged rhyth-mically, seventy times a minute, with a pulse of heightened intensity. The higher the pressure, the greater the stress on the heart—which enlarges progressively to handle the greater de-mand—and on the blood vessels, which initially thicken to withstand the greater pulsation.

After many years, the heart may fail as a pump, unable to maintain the increased work load imposed by the high pressure. As a result of the heart's inability to keep the blood moving forward, fluid begins to accumulate behind the heart; this is congestive heart failure. This fluid squeezed outside of its normal location into various tissues is called *edema*. In the lungs, this edema interferes with breathing and progressive shortness of breath ensues. In the legs, swelling appears.

The repetitive pounding of the high head of pressure against the arterial walls eventually begins to fray the delicate tissues within. Two processes may follow: (1) the vessel may become progressively thinner and thereby susceptible to tearing, allowing blood to escape into the surrounding tissue—the usual cause of a brain hemorrhage, or (2) the vessel may attempt to buffer against the pounding waves by building up various materials within the wall. Unfortunately, these materials include fat and cholesterol and what results is the formation of an atherosclerotic plaque. If the plaque enlarges, it impinges on the flow of blood, leading to an occlusion or thrombosis. Such a process within a coronary artery is responsible for a heart attack.

The Silent Nature of Hypertension

These pressure-induced damages may take many years to lead to a stroke or heart attack. So, for 10, 15, 20 years, hypertension is insidiously causing damage but no symptoms are experienced. It's comparable to the slow buildup of water behind a new dam: not until the water begins to flow over the top may we be aware of the massive accumulation.

Some hypertensives have headaches, dizziness, or nosebleeds, but these are really no more frequent than in people with normal blood pressure. Of course, the pressure may rise to very high levels and cause a hypertensive "crisis," with more severe headaches, mental confusion, and even convulsions, but that picture is fortunately quite rare.

We would all be better off if hypertension hurt a little bit or caused some symptoms that would call attention to its presence.

Thereby, we would be more likely to seek attention, discover the high readings earlier, and do what is needed to bring the pressure down. But as a "silent" process, the only way to identify hypertension before it causes irreparable damage to vital organs is to have a blood pressure reading taken every year.

That sounds simple enough but many do not. A blood pressure check should be part of every contact you make with the health care system: when you see your dentist, your optometrist, or your podiatrist. Your pharmacist may do it but it's more likely he'll provide an automated machine that reads your pressure for fifty cents. Unfortunately, many of these readings are in error but, if we can put men on the moon, we should soon be able to take accurate blood pressure readings automatically.

One way or another, you should have a blood pressure check every year—and in many places free blood pressure checks are available. If the reading is going up and certainly if it's above 140/90, have it rechecked by a physician.

THE TREATMENT OF HYPERTENSION

Although in most cases of hypertension no specific cause can be identified, a number of "secondary" processes can cause the blood pressure to rise (see Table 7).

The most common secondary process is the intake of oral contraceptive pills. Most women who take the pill have a slight rise in blood pressure but that is probably of no consequence. However, about 5 percent will have a rise to above 140/90 after five years of pill use. This problem should be anticipated and a blood pressure taken every six months while using the pill. If the reading has risen it will likely go back down when the pill is stopped.

Most of the other secondary forms of hypertension are associated with some telltale signs, symptoms, or abnormalities appearing in routine laboratory tests such as blood count, urine analysis, and blood chemistry profile. If a warning signal is noted your physician may have more detailed tests performed to determine the diagnosis. The majority of patients

59

Table 7: Secondary Forms of Hypertension

Oral contraceptive pills

Kidney damage

Obstruction of blood flow to the kidneys
(renal vascular hypertension)

Constriction of the aorta (coarctation)

Excess hormones from the adrenal glands
Adrenaline (Pheochromocytoma)
Cortisone (Cushing's disease)
Aldosterone (Primary aldosteronism)

won't need elaborate tests because their hypertension is accompanied by none of these warning signals. But if it is, a further search is worthwhile since most secondary diseases are curable by surgery, such as the repair of a blockage to the kidney artery or removal of an adrenal gland tumor.

Bringing Your Blood Pressure Down

Currently, the chance of curing hypertension by surgery is available for only 5 to 10 percent of hypertensives. The future for the remaining 90 to 95 percent should be brightened by these prospects:

- Your blood pressure may be brought to a safe level without drugs.
- If drugs are needed, they may need to be taken only once a day and without bothersome side effects.
- If your pressure is controlled, you may expect to prevent the development of the cardiovascular complications, thereby living a full and healthy life.

These prospects are much better than those faced by hypertensives just a few years ago. We have made major advances in our understanding of how to manage hypertension, even though we still do not understand its causes.

Nondrug treatment

With or without pills, you should try to lower your blood pressure—and reduce some of the other risks for cardiovascular disease—by these good health habits:

- Shed any excess weight.
- Cut down on the sodium in your diet.
- Follow a regular program of isotonic exercise (see Chapter 8).
- Moderate your alcohol intake.
- Try to relax, with or without a specific relaxation technique.

Neither one nor all of these steps will *necessarily* lower your blood pressure to a safe level, but they will almost certainly help and, at the same time, decrease the risks of obesity, physical inactivity, excess alcohol, and stress. Following a "prudent" diet—low in calories, saturated fat, and sodium—will also help reduce the major risks of a high blood cholesterol.

Proof that these measures will work has come from a five-year test of a group of hypertensive men in Chicago who—rather typically—at the outset evidenced moderate obesity and a slightly elevated blood cholesterol. On a program of diet and exercise—and with no drugs—they were able to achieve and maintain a significant lowering of their blood pressure and serum cholesterol (Table 8).

These healthy habits—along with avoidance of cigarettes—are really what all of us should practice. But those with hypertension have an even greater benefit to be gained: the control of their high blood pressure. Four of these five nondrug treatments are considered in greater detail in subsequent chapters.

61

Table 8: The Results of a Nutritional Exercise Program on 67 Hypertensive Men Overweight at the Onset*

Blood Pressure

YEAR	WEIGHT	SYSTOLIC	DIASTOLIC	SERUM CHOLESTEROL
0	196	147	96	258
1	183	134	86	227
5	186	135	87	233

* From Stamler *et al., JAMA* 243 [1980]: 1819.

We've already covered the problem of dietary sodium but a bit more detail about how to achieve a reasonable and adequate reduction in your sodium intake should be helpful.

Moderate sodium restriction

We're seeking about a 50 percent reduction in your currently excessive (probably) sodium intake. More rigid sodium restriction may be necessary if you have heart failure or other problems, but most of the benefits relative to hypertension can be achieved with a more modest restriction. Not that more rigid restriction would hurt—and if you're able to cut down further, do so. It's just hard to do, unless you go on a diet virtually free of all processed foods, considering the large amount of sodium that's been added to most of them.

The level we're after is about five grams (5,000 milligrams) of sodium chloride a day. Sodium makes up 40 percent of sodium chloride, so that means a two-gram sodium diet. Sodium content is really what we should be considering since sodium salts other than sodium chloride (table salt) are also sources of the sodium that we're trying to reduce.

A number of detailed books are available which you may find useful, including one that's free through your American Heart Association and a number that can be purchased at most bookstores. They contain specific recipes for low-sodium cooking. The free booklet from the American Heart Association is number EM 58 B—"Your Mild Sodium-Restricted Diet," and it contains as much additional information as you'll probably need. But for special recipes you may buy:

"Cooking without Your Salt Shaker" by the American Heart Association, 1978.
Craig Claiborne's Gourmet Diet by C. Claiborne, Times Books, 1980.
The Dieter's Gourmet Cookbook by F. Prince, Cornerstone Library, 1980.
Living with High Blood Pressure by J. D. Margie and J. C. Hunt, HLS Press, 1978.
The Secrets of Salt-Free Cooking by J. Jones, 101 Productions, 1979.

Beyond using these specific recipes, there are really only a few general principles you need to follow to achieve our goal: the two-gram sodium diet shown in Table 9.

1. Be prepared for a bit of a taste letdown for the first few days. A palate that's been overwhelmed by sodium for forty years may take some time to get used to lesser amounts. You may prefer to cut it out gradually, but you'll soon be surprised how much better—and more interesting—many foods taste without the sodium. And after you've killed the salt habit, you'll probably cringe when you inadvertently come across a high-sodium food. You'll wonder how you ever loved mother's chicken soup.

2. Add no table salt in the cooking or at the table. If you need seasoning, choose one from the bottom of Table 9. But avoid garlic salt, onion salt, celery salt, seasoned salt, sea salt, soy sauce, Teriyaki sauce,

Table 9: A Two-Gram Sodium Diet

	Foods You May Eat	Foods You Should Not Eat
Beverages	2 cups per day of whole milk, skim milk, chocolate milk Coffee, tea, decaffeinated beverages, carbonated beverages (coke)	Buttermilk, tomato juice, V-8 juice
Bread	3 slices of regular bread All other breads must be: Low-sodium bread Low-sodium crackers Commercial corn tortillas	All other breads Regular saltine crackers
Cereal	½ cup regular cooked cereal without salt, puffed rice, puffed wheat, and shredded wheat	Instant and quick cooking cereals All other dry cereals
Dessert	1 serving: cake, cookies, or puddings made with milk allowance and sodium-free leavening agents Unsalted fruit pie Gelatin desserts made with plain gelatin and foods allowed	All other commercially prepared desserts
Fat	¼ cup cream Regular margarine (3 tbsp. per day) Low-sodium salad dressing	Commercial mayonnaise and salad dressing All others
Fruit	4 (½ cup) servings: fruit juices, nectars;	Salted tomato juice, frozen apples,

Table 9—Continued

	Foods You May Eat	Foods You Should Not Eat
& fruit juice	all fresh, frozen, or canned fruit Dried dates or prunes	casaba melon, all other dried fruits
Meat & eggs	Broiled, fried, roasted, or stewed beef, veal, pork, lamb, poultry, freshwater fish, cod, flounder, haddock, halibut, mackeral, perch, salt-free (dietetic) canned salmon and tuna, lobster, oysters (limit 5), calf and chicken liver, low-sodium cheese	All cheese except cottage Barbecued, breaded, canned, cured, and smoked meats or fish Frankfurters, luncheon meat, ham, bacon, sausage
Soup	Unsalted broth Commercial low-sodium soups	All commercially prepared soups and instant mixes
Sweets	Chocolate, cocoa, honey, white sugar 1 tsp. jam, jelly, or preserves	Commercial candy, molasses, syrup, Dutch-process cocoa
Vegetables	All fresh, frozen, or dietetic (low-salt) canned vegetables	All regularly canned vegetables Potato chips (Fritos, Doritos, etc.) Sauerkraut, pickles
Miscellaneous	Dry mustard, fresh garlic, lemon juice, pepper, vinegar, yeast Unsalted popcorn Salt-free baking powder, ¼ cup cornmeal	Baking powder, celery seeds, parsley, salt, *soda*, all seasoned salts, self-rising cornmeal and flour Sauces containing salt

Table 9—Continued

	Foods You May Eat	Foods You Should Not Eat
Miscel-laneous (continued)	Cornstarch, 2 tbsp. flour, unsalted peanut butter	such as catsup, chili sauce, soy sauce, steak sauces, prepared horseradish, prepared mustard, meat tenderizer
		Olives, pickles, salted nuts
		Salted popcorn, pretzels, TV dinners, ACCENT

Instead of salt (sodium) you may improve the taste of many foods by using these herbs and spices:

Allspice	Ginger	Pimiento
Basil	Lemon	Poppy seed
Bay leaf	Marjoram	Rosemary
Caraway seed	Mint	Saffron
Cardamon	Mustard (dry)	Sage
*Chili powder	Nutmeg	Savory
Chives	*Onion or	Sesame seed
Cinnamon	onion powder	Tarragon
Cloves	Oregano	Thyme
Cumin	Paprika	Turmeric
Curry powder	Parsley (fresh)	
Dill	Pepper	
*Garlic or	(red, green,	
garlic powder	black, white)	

---

* These 3 are particularly useful:

Chili powder on beef, eggs, corn, eggplant, lima beans, onions, Spanish sauces, tomatoes

Garlic or garlic powder (but not garlic salt) on fish, meats, salads, soups, tomatoes

Onion or onion powder (but not onion salt) on meats, salads, vegetables

MSG, Worcestershire sauce, bouillon cubes —they are full of sodium.

3. Unless you have a kidney disease, you may try salt substitutes which contain potassium, which may be helpful particularly if you're also taking a diuretic pill which tends to remove potassium from your body. Some find pure potassium substitutes (such as Co-Salt, Neocurtasol) somewhat bitter. A reasonable alternative—for the little bit of salt you need—is Morton's Lite-Salt, half sodium and half potassium.

4. Avoid most canned foods since they have had sodium added in the processing. If you use them, drain off the liquid.

5. Most fresh-frozen foods are low in sodium but check the label to see if any has been added. Though a few of the low-sodium cookbooks advise that you avoid some fresh "high-sodium" vegetables (beets, carrots, celery, spinach, turnips) that's not really necessary because they aren't actually "high-sodium."

6. On the other hand, avoid all pickled vegetables and meats. One green olive has almost 100 milligrams of sodium—more than a cup of beets. One medium dill pickle has almost 1000 milligrams of sodium, half of a full day's supply. As an alternative to these salt mines, use fresh cauliflower or tomatoes or just about any unpickled vegetable.

7. Be careful about intake of milk and cheeses. One ounce of whole milk has about 125 milligrams of sodium and most natural cheeses about 200 milligrams per ounce. Processed American or Swiss cheese has almost 400 milligrams per ounce. Low-sodium cheeses are available.

8. Fresh water should be no problem even in some areas where well water contains a fair amount of sodium. You can hardly drink enough water to get too much sodium from it. But club soda contains from 20 to 40 milligrams per 8-ounce bottle, and you should watch out for bottled mineral waters as well.

9. Beware of some other hidden sources of sodium, including such popular antacids as Alka-Seltzer (521 milligrams of sodium per dose), Bromo-Seltzer (717 mg), Sal Hepatica (1,000 mg), and Bi-So-Gel (420 mg). On the other hand, Maalox, Di-gel, Rolaids, and Riopan are quite low in sodium.

10. And lastly, watch out for most fast foods (see Table 10, "The Sodium Content of Some Fast Foods"). Somebody told me the least salty food at McDonald's was the French fries. At regular restaurants, ask for food prepared without lots of sodium, such as individually prepared fish or steak, fresh vegetables, vinegar-and-oil salad dressing, and fresh fruit.

11. When all is said and done, never say never. You certainly may enjoy any food regardless of high sodium content—even anchovies —on occasion. Just try to be good to yourself most of the time. Remember, eat more fresh foods, meats, vegetables, and fruits.

The value of other nondrug therapies

Though a good deal more will be said about weight reduction, exercise, alcohol, and relief of stress in subsequent chapters, a few additional comments about their specific effects on the blood pressure seem in order.

Weight reduction will almost always lower an elevated

Table 10: The Sodium Content of Some Fast Foods

Item	Average Sodium Content (mgs per portion)
HAMBURGERS	
Burger King Whopper	990
Jack-in-the-Box Jumbo	1010
McDonald's Big Mac	960
BEEF SANDWICHES	
Arby's Roast Beef	870
Burger King Chopped Steak	965
Roy Rogers Roast Beef	610
FISH	
Arthur Treacher's	420
Burger King	970
Long John Silver	1335
McDonald's	710
CHICKEN	
Kentucky Fried 3-Piece Dinner	2285
OTHER SPECIALTY ITEMS	
Jack-in-the-Box Taco Meal	925
Pizza Hut Pizza Supreme	1280
Wendy's Chili	1190

blood pressure, about one millimeter of pressure for each two pounds in weight. Though additional benefits may result from the combination of a decreased sodium intake with the reduced calories, the fall in blood pressure seems to relate directly to the weight loss.

Regular exercise may be associated with a fall in blood pressure, but it is uncertain if this is an effect of the exercise itself. Most who begin a regular, intensive exercise program lose weight, change their diets, and quit smoking. Regardless of why it happens, the end result is helpful. But a word of caution: the blood pressure rises markedly during isometric or static exercise. Since we shall see that this form of exercise is of little benefit, you should not do isometrics.

Moderate alcohol intake, one to two ounces of ethanol per day, may be helpful for cardiovascular health but excessive drinking is associated with higher blood pressure and more cardiovascular disease. For now, let's simply say, "As in all things, moderation."

Relaxation by virtually any technique will lower the blood pressure during the period of relaxation. The pressure falls as much as 40 mm Hg during sleep. But with rare exceptions, the effect has not been shown to persist between periods of relaxation or after a program has been completed. If you want to use one or another relaxation technique, feel free to do so. It may reduce your pressure, but don't depend upon it.

Drugs to Lower Your Blood Pressure

Even if you follow all of the nondrug therapies, your blood pressure may not come down or stay down to a safe level. Or you may be unwilling to make the changes in diet and lifestyle that are needed to make them work. Either way, the chances are that you will need to take one or more pills each day for your hypertension. If so, these general guidelines should be followed:

1. Your therapy will almost certainly be lifelong. Rarely do patients with essential hypertension get over their hypertension unless they shed some aggravating factor, such as obesity or the use of estrogens. Keep taking your pills, even if you feel perfectly well, *particularly* if you feel perfectly well.

2. The goal of therapy is keeping your blood pressure below 140/90, preferably near 120/80. Less rigorous control may be acceptable if you have certain problems with more vigorous treatment.

3. You should have your pressure checked every few months even after you achieve good control. Something may happen to change your pressure. Don't be concerned if it fluctuates some between visits; a change of as much as 20 mm Hg may reflect nothing more than temporary stress or natural variation.

4. You should anticipate the possibility of occasional, temporary side effects. Any therapy that significantly lowers your pressure may cause you to feel tired and weak temporarily. All therapies may produce some side effects, as will be described later. If you don't feel well, don't just stop the therapy and skip your next appointment. Discuss the situation with your doctor. Tell him or her what's bothering you. Changes in your therapy can almost always be made to overcome any bothersome side effects. Remember, the alternative to therapy is worse— incapacity or premature death.

5. Recognize that it's going to cost from ten cents to as much as three dollars a day for your drugs. This may seem expensive but, again, remember the alternatives.

6. Be sure you understand your doctor's directions about the types of medications (each should be labeled), the time of day to take them, the precautions about side effects, and so on. Different drugs are used according to different schedules, some once a day, others as often as four times a day.

7. Don't forget to take your medication as directed. If you take one pill a day, take it immediately upon awakening, or when you brush your teeth. If you take three or four a day, take them before or after meals. Get into the habit of taking your pills routinely at the same time so you don't forget. It's easy to forget, particularly when you feel well. Many who take multiple doses of one or more pills a day put a day's supply into a little pillbox and carry that with them at all times, so they'll never be caught short.

8. Don't give up if you happen to miss a dose or two, but don't take all the doses you've missed at one time to make up the losses. Just get back on the prescribed schedule.

9. Don't worry about becoming dependent on a drug or embarrassed that your health depends upon some pill. Having hypertension is no sign of weakness or inadequacy. Having hypertension and not treating it *is* a sign of weakness and maybe even stupidity.

10. Don't take other medications without telling your doctor. You may interfere with the control of your hypertension or bring on unnecessary side effects. As an example, diet pills for weight reduction may block the effects of certain antihypertensives. When you stop the diet pills, your blood pressure may then suddenly fall too low.

The types of drugs

There are three main classes of drugs now being used to treat hypertension. They are:

1. Diuretics.
2. Sympathetic nervous inhibitors.
3. Vasodilators.

Their mode of action is shown in Figure 9. In the untreated state, your blood pressure is elevated because the vessels are tight and the volume of blood within them may be increased.

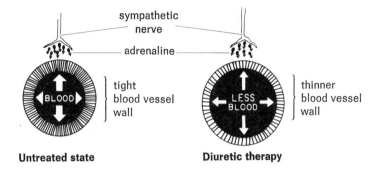

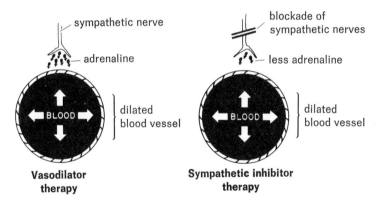

Figure 9. A stylized representation of the effects of the three major types of antihypertensive medications upon the blood pressure. The untreated state (upper left) involves an overfilled, tight circulation. With diuretic therapy (upper right), excess sodium and fluid are excreted, reducing the amount in the circulation and thinning the blood vessel walls. With vasodilator therapy (lower left), the vessel walls are directly dilated. With sympathetic blocking drugs (lower right), the vessels dilate because they are relieved of some of the constriction previously caused by activity of the sympathetic nerves through the hormone adrenalin.

73

The tightening may reflect the action of adrenaline, a hormone released from the adrenal glands and the sympathetic nerves, the nerves which automatically regulate various body functions such as heartbeat and breathing. Even if there is no excess of sympathetic nervous function, decreasing the activity of the sympathetic nerves will relax the blood vessels.

Under diuretic therapy, the diuretics lower your blood pressure by increasing the flow of urine, removing some of the fluid from the overfilled circulation, and ridding some of the sodium and water from the blood vessel walls, making them less tight.

A number of drugs decrease the activity of the sympathetic nerves. Though these drugs act in different places within the body, their end result is to inhibit the sympathetic nerves partially and thereby allow the blood vessels to dilate.

The third category of drugs, vasodilators, acts directly upon the blood vessel walls to cause them to dilate.

These drugs are most often used in a stepwise sequence, a diuretic first, then a sympathetic inhibitor, and then a vasodilator. About half of all hypertensives will have their pressure brought under good control with just a diuretic. The other half will need two or more drugs. If you need more than one drug, don't assume that your hypertension is necessarily more severe. Different people with similar levels of blood pressure may respond differently to some medications. Don't expect your pressure to respond in the same manner as other hypertensives. And it follows that you shouldn't take another person's drugs without your doctor's consent.

Regardless of which drug you take, bothersome side effects may develop. Some are more common with certain drugs but fatigue, loss of mental alertness and, in men, decrease in sexual potency are the most frequent. If anything unusual develops, discuss the situation with your physician. You and your physician should be able to work out a regimen that will control your blood pressure without bothersome side effects. The trouble it takes to do so is certainly worthwhile since, by controlling your hypertension, you will live longer and better.

FIVE

Cholesterol and Saturated Fat

An elevated blood cholesterol is the third major risk factor for cardiovascular disease. This risk may be even more common than ordinarily considered because most Americans may have too high a level of cholesterol, even though it's not above what is considered "normal." To illustrate the meaning of "normal," let us compare the curves of the serum cholesterol in the population of south Japan and east Finland (Figure 10). Notice that the average level in the Japanese is about 140, whereas it's twice as high, almost 300, in the Finnish people. What is significant about these figures is that the death rate from coronary heart disease in Finland is the world's highest, almost 900 per 100,000, while the Japanese have the world's lowest, 102 per 100,000 (Figure 11). In the United States, the average serum cholesterol is about halfway between the Japanese and the Finnish, about 220 mg, and we have a mortality rate from heart attacks of 670 per 100,000, closer to the Finns than the Japanese.

These figures suggest that our current epidemic of heart disease may be related to a "normal" serum cholesterol that is actually undesirably high. Obviously, what is considered "normal," because it's "usual," may not be normal at all. In a tribe of pygmies, being four feet tall may be considered "nor-

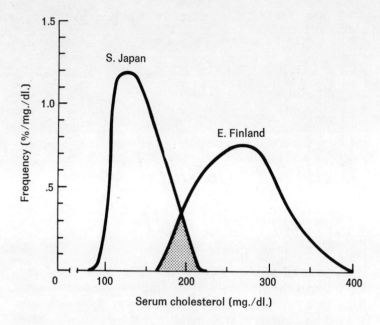

Figure 10. The frequency distribution of serum cholesterol in a representative sample of people in south Japan and east Finland.

mal." With our "normal" cholesterol, we have a great amount of heart disease and the two may be directly related.

THE RISK OF
HIGH BLOOD CHOLESTEROL

The cholesterol-heart disease relationship is suggested by the results of a carefully controlled, five-year study in Norway.[1] More than one thousand healthy Norwegian men, aged 40 to 49 with moderately high blood cholesterol levels, were randomly divided into two groups. Half, the control group, were left alone. The other half, the intervention group, were asked

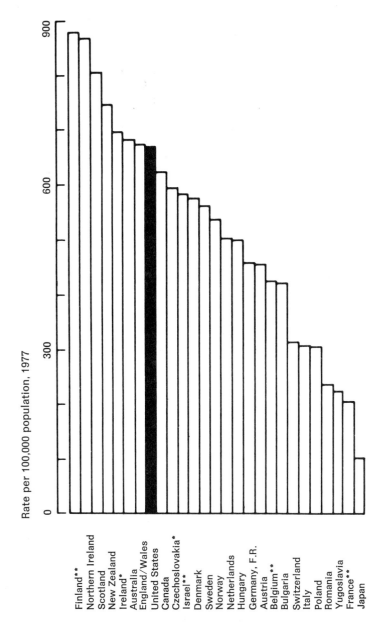

Figure 11. Death rates from coronary heart disease in 25 countries for men aged 35 to 74. Those with * are for 1975, those with ** are for 1976, the others are for 1977. (Source: Levy, R. I., "Declining Mortality in Coronary Heart Disease," *Arteriosclerosis* 1 [1981]: 314. By permission of the American Heart Association, Inc.)

to follow a diet with fewer saturated fats and slightly more polyunsaturated fats. Those on the diet were also asked to stop smoking.

At the end of five years, the men on the diet had the expected decrease in their average blood cholesterol level, from 328 milligrams (per 100 milliliters) to 263, whereas the average cholesterol level of the control men actually rose slightly, from 328 to 341. Along with this fall in cholesterol, the 604 on the diet suffered significantly less sudden cardiovascular disease and death than did the 628 in the control group.

Beyond the consistent relation between levels of blood cholesterol and the frequency of coronary heart disease,[2] there's a great deal of additional evidence incriminating cholesterol as an important risk for atherosclerosis:

- Cholesterol is the predominant fatty material within the atherosclerotic plaques responsible for most heart disease.
- The unfortunate people who inherit a very high cholesterol have heart disease at a very early age, some dying of heart attacks in their early teens.
- Animals fed high cholesterol diets develop atherosclerosis and heart disease; when the diet is changed and the blood cholesterol is allowed to fall, the atherosclerosis recedes.

These facts point to a direct relationship between increased levels of blood cholesterol and the development of atherosclerosis and heart disease. The therapeutic trial from Norway is additional evidence, showing that, by lowering the cholesterol level, the frequency of heart disease can be lowered.

All of these points have been put together into a Diet-Heart model to explain the high prevalence of atherosclerotic heart disease in most Western, industrialized countries (Figure 12). The combination of what we eat and our heredity leads to increased blood cholesterol (hypercholesterolemia), the first stage. This in turn, aggravated by the presence of hypertension,

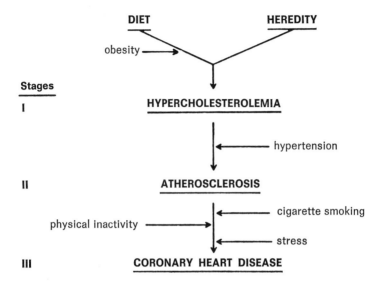

Figure 12. The "Diet-Heart" model, relating the development of coronary heart disease to the combination of diet and heredity.

leads to stage 2, atherosclerosis, which, when accelerated by cigarette smoking, physical inactivity, and stress, leads to coronary heart disease.

Most medical researchers accept this model, though some do not believe the circumstantial evidence provides proof of a cause-and-effect relationship. These skeptics have been particularly bothered by the lack of proof, in man, that lowering the cholesterol level resulted in a definite reduction in atherosclerosis or heart disease. The positive results of the Norwegian trial should reduce some of this skepticism.

HOW DOES OUR DIET
LEAD TO HIGH CHOLESTEROL?

The diet-heart model starts with a combination of diet and heredity. The component of our diet that seems responsible is the fat, specifically that which is "saturated." The term *saturated* refers to the chemical nature of those fats which are of animal origin and are almost always solid at room temperatures. In various populations, the death rate from cardiovascular disease relates directly to the amount of saturated fat in the diet.

This saturated fat is the source of most of the cholesterol in the blood. The liver is an efficient converter of dietary fat into cholesterol. On the other hand, some of the cholesterol eaten (as in egg yolks) may also be absorbed and contribute to the pool of cholesterol in the body. Some of us absorb much of this preformed cholesterol, others little at all.

On the other hand, those fats that are unsaturated tend to reduce the amount of cholesterol made in the liver. The more unsaturated or polyunsaturated, the better. These unsaturated fats are present in vegetables and almost all are liquid at room temperatures. Thus, diets used to lower the level of blood cholesterol usually combine a decrease in saturated (animal) fat with an increase in polyunsaturated (vegetable) oil.

GOOD AND BAD CHOLESTEROL

Until a few years ago, all cholesterol was considered bad, other than for the small amount needed in various critical body functions. The cholesterol in blood, being relatively insoluble in plasma, is known to travel attached to various proteins, called lipoproteins, which keep it dissolved in the blood. When the total cholesterol was broken down into its various lipoprotein components, some very interesting relationships began to emerge:

- Most cholesterol is carried on a lipoprotein that is of low density (low-density lipoprotein or LDL) because of its larger size. The LDL cholesterol is the form which is made in the liver, enters the blood, gets into cells, and builds up atherosclerotic plaques. The higher the LDL cholesterol, the more heart disease.

· About one-fourth of blood cholesterol is carried on a lipoprotein of smaller size or higher density (high-density lipoprotein or HDL) which transports the cholesterol out of the tissues to the liver where it is broken down and excreted into the bile. This is the good cholesterol: the higher the HDL cholesterol, the less heart disease.

A variety of circumstances wherein heart disease didn't seem to relate to total cholesterol have now been shown to relate to the level of HDL cholesterol. As examples:

· Consumption of moderate amounts of alcohol has been shown to reduce the rate of cardiovascular deaths. These amounts of alcohol clearly raise the level of HDL cholesterol.
· Strenuous exercise raises HDL cholesterol.
· Women before menopause who have less atherosclerosis and heart disease have higher HDL levels (to live the longest: be a woman who jogs to the liquor store every day).
· Cigarette smokers and obese people, at higher risk for heart disease, have lower HDL levels.

And so the story goes: high HDL cholesterol appears to offer protection against atherosclerosis, presumably by keeping cholesterol out of the blood vessel walls. And, as you might expect, diets high in saturated fats tend to raise the bad LDL, diets high in polyunsaturated fats tend to raise the good HDL.

You may have heard about another measure of the fat (lipid) content of blood, the level of plasma *triglycerides*. If these are very, very high, they may themselves induce trouble.

But moderately high triglycerides don't seem to be an independent risk factor. They frequently accompany a high total cholesterol or low HDL cholesterol, and it's these latter levels that seem to be the culprits.

HOW TO ACHIEVE A LOWER FAT DIET

Our objective is to achieve the Revised U. S. Dietary Goals (Figure 13), goals that seem sensible, feasible, and in keeping with the "prudent diet" proposed by the American Heart

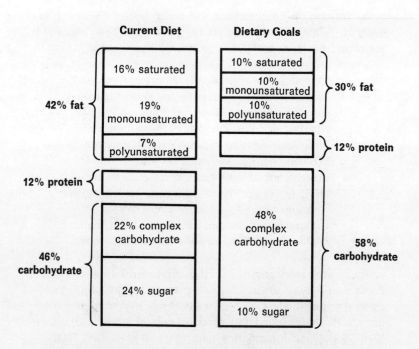

Figure 13. A breakdown of the components of the average current American diet and the Revised U.S. Dietary Goals advocated by the Senate Select Committee on Nutrition and Human Needs in 1978.

Association and experts in England and Scandinavia. Although the reduction in total fat from the 42 percent in our current average diet to 30 percent is less than that advocated by Pritikin and others, it seems to be as much as most of us are willing and able to achieve. Moreover, on the basis of studies such as the Norwegian trial, such a level would be adequate to reduce the burden of high blood cholesterol for most of us. For some with a very high cholesterol, a more stringent diet may be needed, along with drugs that further reduce the blood cholesterol level.

The general approach is to reduce or virtually eliminate as many high-fat foods as possible and increase the quantity of foods of low-fat content (see Table 11, "The Basics of the Prudent Diet"). What you should be after is not some rapid effect from a short-term "crash" diet but a gradual, permanent change in your eating habits. It should not be looked upon as a punishment, but rather an attractive and acceptable alternative to what you are now eating. To follow such a diet, these guidelines should be helpful:

1. Cut down on red meat, and that meat which is eaten should be lean. Veal is better than most beef or pork cuts but is less helpful than poultry (other than duck) and fish.

2. Get rid of as much visible fat as possible before cooking and certainly before eating. This includes chicken skins—although even the most dedicated eater likely will give in occasionally to crispy "Kentucky fried."

3. Broil or roast meats, poultry, and fish, allowing the fat to drip off—do not collect for gravies. If you make a gravy from the pan juices, it is best to chill it and skim off the fat that floats to the top or use a cup that has a spout that starts at the bottom and leaves the fatty portion on top.

4. Cut down on organ meats (liver, brains, sweetbreads) and egg yolks, which are very

Table 11: The Basics of the Prudent Diet*

Food Group	Recommended	Avoid or Use Sparingly
Meat Poultry Fish	Chicken, turkey, veal, fish	Duck, goose
	Shellfish: clams, crab, lobster, oysters, scallops	Shrimp
Dried beans and peas		
Nuts		
Eggs	Beef, lamb, pork, ham less frequently	Heavily marbled and fatty meats, spare ribs, mutton, sausages, frank-furters, fatty ham-burgers, bacon, luncheon meats
		Organ meats (liver, kidney, heart, sweetbread)
Vegetables and fruits	Any fresh or frozen vegetables or fruits (preferable to canned or otherwise processed, which often have extra sodium)	If you must limit your calories, use higher calorie vegetables such as potatoes, corn, and lima beans sparingly
Breads and cereals	Breads made with a minimum of saturated fat: white enriched,	Butter rolls, com-mercial biscuits, doughnuts, sweet

* Adapted from *Heartbook* by the American Heart Association. Copyright © 1980 American Heart Association. Reprinted by permission of the publisher, E. P. Dutton, Inc.

Table 11—Continued

Food Group	Recommended	Avoid or Use Sparingly
Breads and cereals (continued)	whole wheat, muffins, french bread, pumpernickel, rye bread, homemade biscuits, muffins, and griddle cakes (using an allowed liquid oil as shortening)	rolls, cakes, crackers, egg bread, cheese bread, commercial mixes containing dried eggs and whole milk
	Cereals (hot and cold), rice, melba toast, matzo, pretzels	
	Pasta: macaroni, noodles (except egg noodles), spaghetti	
Milk products	Milk products that are low in dairy fats: skim (nonfat) milk, low-fat milk, buttermilk made from skim milk, yogurt made from skim milk, canned evaporated skim milk, cocoa made with low-fat milk	Whole milk and whole milk products: chocolate milk, canned whole milk, ice cream, all creams including sour, half-and-half, and whipped; whole milk yogurt
		Nondairy cream substitutes (usually contain coconut oil)

Table 11—Continued

Food Group	Recommended	Avoid or Use Sparingly
Milk products (continued)		Cheese made from cream or whole milk
		Butter
Fats and oils	Margarines, liquid oil shortenings, salad dressings and mayonnaise containing any of these polyunsaturated vegetable oils: corn oil, cottonseed oil, safflower oil, sesame seed oil, soybean oil, sunflower seed oil	Solid fats and shortenings: butter, lard, salt pork fat, meat fat, completely hydrogenated margarines and vegetable shortenings, products containing coconut oil
	Margarines and other products high in polyunsaturates	
Other foods to meet energy needs	Low in calories or no calories:	Coconut and coconut oil, commercial cakes, pies, cookies and mixes, frozen cream pies, commercially fried such as potato chips and other deep-fried snacks,
	Fresh fruit or fruit canned without sugar, tea, coffee (no cream), cocoa powder, water ices, gelatin, fruit whip, puddings made with nonfat milk,	

Table 11—Continued

Food Group	Recommended	Avoid or Use Sparingly
Other foods to meet energy needs (continued)	low-calorie drinks, vinegar, mustard, ketchup, herbs, spices High in calories: Frozen or canned fruit with sugar added, jelly, jam, marmalade, honey, pure sugar candy, cakes, pies, cookies, puddings made with polyunsaturated fat, angel food cake, nuts, especially walnuts, peanut butter, bottled drinks, fruit drinks, ice milk, sherbert, wine, beer, whiskey	whole milk puddings, chocolate pudding, ice cream

high in cholesterol. As noted earlier, you may not absorb much of this preformed cholesterol but there's no way to know if you do or do not. It is safer to reduce your cholesterol consumption and not to worry.

5. Use low-fat (1 to 2 percent butterfat) or skim (0.5 percent) milk instead of regular whole milk (3.5 percent). Buttermilk (despite its name) is okay, as is low-fat yogurt. Most ice creams have 10 percent fat, some, such as Haagen-Dazs and Baskin-Robbins, even more.

Try ice milk or sherbet instead. Watch out for processed cream substitutes for your coffee—most are full of coconut oil, which, although of vegetable origin, is one of the most saturated fats of all. And be careful about most hard and processed cheeses; they may be 40 percent butterfat.

6. Substitute polyunsaturated vegetable oils (safflower and corn) and soft margarines (Mazola or Fleishmann's) for butter, lard, and chicken fat. But limit your use of olive oil and watch out for the worst of all, coconut oil and palm oils.

7. For desserts, cut down on chocolate and all those rich, creamy, gooey delicacies. Fresh fruits are best (except for avocado) and most nuts are okay.

When less saturated fat (especially meat) is eaten, the diet almost certainly will be higher in fiber from unrefined cereal grains and raw vegetables. Fiber is vegetable matter that resists digestion and includes several different substances. We are now eating in our typical diet only about one-third of the amount of fiber people were eating in 1900, when there was less heart disease and cancer. The low incidence of both colon cancer and heart disease seen among the Japanese may reflect the higher fiber content of their diet.

There's no doubt that increasing the amount of fiber in the diet will increase the size and softness of the stool, offering some protection from constipation, hemorrhoids, and diverticulosis (and likely increase abdominal gas). But along with the bulk, the fiber may trap some of the fat, cholesterol, and other harmful substances that are eaten or secreted into the gut.

To add more fiber to your diet, eat more whole grains and raw, unpeeled fruits and vegetables. High-fiber grain foods include bran and wheat cereals, rye bread, whole wheat bread, corn, graham crackers, oats, popcorn, brown rice, and spaghetti.

Fruits rich in fiber include apples, oranges, pears, and strawberries. Some high-fiber vegetables are beans, beets, broccoli, celery, kale greens, peas, and squash.

In following any of the diets mentioned in this book—low in sodium, calories, or saturated fat—it would be helpful to know what's in the processed foods that many of us depend on (see Chapter 4). Current regulations demand only that all ingredients in processed foods be listed in the order of their quantity, by weight. When you see "salt" as the second ingredient you can be reasonably sure there is a lot more of it than when it's listed as the ninth ingredient. But you really can't tell how much salt you're getting in either situation. A bit more information is provided about the type of fat or shortening present. To reduce your intake of saturated fats, avoid foods listing fat as a major ingredient, particularly if it's animal fat (butter or lard), hydrogenated vegetable oil, coconut oil, or palm oil. Be careful about "vegetable oil," since that could be one of the saturated ones. Manufacturers are beginning to provide more complete information on ingredients, but they still have a long way to go before it will be really helpful to consumers.

Some excellent sources of imaginative, tasty recipes that are low in fat (and therefore low in calories and many also low in sodium) are:

The American Heart Association Cookbook (David McKay, 1979).

Living Better—Recipes for a Healthy Heart by J. D. Margie, R. L. Levy, and J. C. Hunt (HLS Press, 1981).

Craig Claiborne's Gourmet Diet by C. Claiborne (Times Books, 1980).

The Dieter's Gourmet Cookbook by F. Prince (Cornerstone Library, 1980).

The Need to Start Early

High blood cholesterols and coronary arteries full of cholesterol-containing plaques are found in many Americans in their teens and twenties. We need to start early to avoid such trouble and to establish good eating habits that will be carried on for a lifetime of better health.

So first, keep your child slim. Childhood obesity sets the stage for much lifelong obesity. Today's pediatricians are advising parents to start infants on the way to a life free of cardiovascular disease in the following ways:

1. Breast milk is best and solid foods should not be started until the child is four to six months old. Add no sodium to any baby food and avoid those processed ones with added sodium.
2. Provide only a reasonable amount of food, as judged mainly by a steady and appropriate weight gain. If baby is getting pudgy, cut down the amount and richness of the foods.
3. Avoid rich, creamy foods and those full of sugar or salt. Candy and ice cream should be avoided.
4. After the first year, use low-fat or skim milk and follow the general principles of the prudent diet.

    Along with lots of exercise, such diet practices should help establish a healthy lifelong trimness and avoidance of extra calories, saturated fats, and sodium.

As children grow into their teens, they should be encouraged to continue good dietary practices. One of the most important principles is to insist on three "square meals" a day, including a balanced breakfast. Children whose breakfast staples are cokes and doughnuts are malnourished. And keep nutritious, low-fat foods around for snacks.

There's obviously a great deal more about proper nutrition than can be covered here. In addition to the books of recipes mentioned here and in Chapter 4, Jane Brody's *Nutrition Book*

(W. W. Norton, 1981) is a 552-page gold mine of good information. However, most of what you need to know is provided in this book. Don't be misled by claims for weird diets and supplements. You don't have to become a vegetarian—though if you did, it wouldn't hurt. The prudent diet has been proven to work and to be safe. On the other hand, keep an open mind: garlic has also been shown to lower the cholesterol levels.

And if you follow the prudent diet and thereby control your cholesterol level, think of the extra satisfaction you will have knowing that occasionally it's okay to lay one on—have a six-course banquet at the best French restaurant in town to celebrate your anniversary. Enjoy the rich dressings, sauces, and desserts because, as long as it's an infrequent occasion, your regular, prudent diet is protecting your blood vessels and heart. Those gluttons who eat such rich food regularly not only lose the satisfaction of enjoying a special treat but they will almost certainly not be around long enough to enjoy many more.

SIX

Obesity

While much of the world is starving, most Americans are eating too much: obesity is the American brand of malnutrition. And would you believe—despite our compulsive fixation on dieting and exercising to lose weight—the average weight of American adults has continued to increase. In 1980, the typical American was ten to twenty pounds above the "ideal" weight.

As we shall see, this amount of excess weight is more of a social problem than a medical disease. Though anything beyond 25 percent above the "ideal" is very likely to be harmful, most of us who are ten to twenty pounds overweight are not endangering our health—from the weight itself. If the excess weight is accompanied by high blood cholesterol, hypertension, or diabetes, as it often is, then it is a problem. However, by itself, without these accompanying risk factors, a little bit of excess weight is not harmful.

To keep matters straight, let's use these definitions: *overweight* is anything from 1 percent to 19 percent more than the desirable weight; *obesity* is more than 20 percent above this weight. Since height obviously is important in deciding what is the normal weight, the best indicator of body weight is the "body mass index" (BMI), which is derived by dividing the weight by the square of the height. Referring to Figure 14,

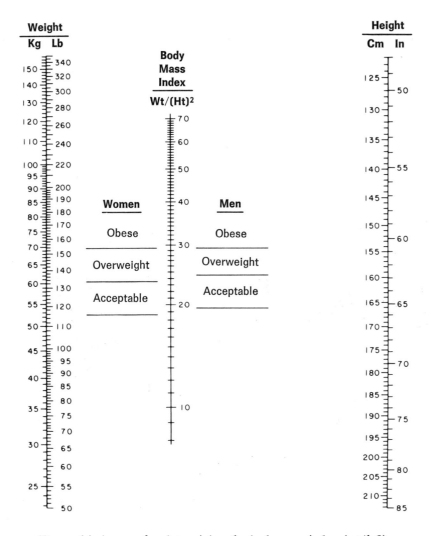

Figure 14. A score for determining the body mass index (wt/ht²). Place a ruler between the body weight (left-hand column) and the height (right-hand column) using either the metric or avoirdupois scales. The body mass index is the point where the line connecting the weight and height crosses the body mass index column in the middle. (Source: copyright 1978 George A. Bray, M.D.)

93

place a ruler across your weight and height (using either the metric or avoirdupois measures) and determine your BMI. If you are above 25, you are overweight; about 30 and you're obese. We will mainly consider those who are truly obese because they make up a sizable number of people and they are at increased risk of heart disease.

THE RISKS OF OBESITY

The causes of the excess mortality associated with obesity include coronary artery disease (sudden death and angina), hypertension, and diabetes. In fact, obese people have a higher death rate from virtually all causes of death except suicide. An obvious rejoinder to that fact is that their continued eating is a form of suicide, so that the really fat are in trouble from every direction.

"Morbid" Obesity

When obesity becomes severe—or as it is aptly termed, "morbid"—death and debilitating disease occur at very high rates. This degree of obesity is usually defined as over 50 percent above average weight. In one study of 200 such morbidly obese men in Los Angeles, Dr. E. J. Drenick and his coworkers observed that the death rate was twelve times above average for the younger, 25- to 34-year-old men and three times above average for 45- to 54-year-old men. Their deaths were mostly from cardiovascular disease. Since they died at such an early age, fewer lived long enough to develop cancer.

There are about 1 million of these morbidly obese people in the United States. Their very high risks for serious trouble has led to such drastic treatments as intestinal bypass operations and prolonged periods of total starvation.

"Moderate" Obesity

At least three of the clearly defined risk factors for preventable heart disease frequently accompany moderate obesity (20 percent to 40 percent overweight)—elevated blood cholesterol, hypertension, and diabetes. Among the obese people in the Framingham study, not only did the total cholesterol levels tend to be high but there were lower levels of the "good" type of cholesterol, the high-density lipoprotein (HDL) form which was noted in Chapter 5, to protect against atherosclerosis. Fortunately, if such people lose weight, the levels of HDL cholesterol usually rise, which is probably responsible for some of the lowering of their cardiovascular risk that accompanies weight loss.

Hypertension is at least twice as common among people who are 20 percent or more above normal weight. Though hypertension does not develop in every obese person, there is a general relation: the greater the weight gain, the higher the blood pressure. How this comes about is unknown though there appears to be a retention of extra sodium, possibly related to some of the hormonal abnormalities that accompany weight gain. As noted in Chapter 4, sodium retention may be the primary disturbance behind most hypertension, so the connection between weight gain and blood pressure is a logical one.

Those who are fat will usually have a fall in blood pressure if they lose weight and this should be the first treatment attempted for hypertension. Even more importantly, the prevention of obesity may prevent the development of hypertension. As shown in a long-term study of high school students in Pittsburgh, those teenage boys who gained the most weight tended to have the highest blood pressures.

The last of the three probable mechanisms for the greater risk for cardiovascular disease is the frequent association of obesity and diabetes, which almost always accelerates the development of atherosclerosis. Even without obvious diabetes, most obese people have other disturbances in the way they handle sugar—abnormal glucose tolerance—which may provoke cardiovascular trouble.

"Minimal" Obesity

We've seen that obesity is frequently accompanied by major risk factors for heart disease and that the relief of obesity may help relieve these risks. But do the "minimally" obese (body weight 10 percent to 20 percent above normal) have increased risk even if they don't have accompanying high cholesterol, hypertension, or diabetes? The answer that most of you—and most doctors—would likely give is yes. Statements such as "obesity is the number one health problem today" continue to appear in medical journals and are probably responsible for part of our national obsession with obesity.

But recent evidence has tended to deny that the excess ten

Table 12: Average Weights for Men and Women*

Average Weights for Men 25 and Over
(weight in pounds, in indoor clothing)

HEIGHT (SHOES ON 1" HEELS)	SMALL FRAME	MEDIUM FRAME	LARGE FRAME
5'2"	112–120	118–129	126–141
5'3"	115–123	121–133	129–144
5'4"	118–126	124–136	132–148
5'5"	121–129	127–139	135–152
5'6"	124–133	130–143	138–156
5'7"	128–137	134–147	142–161
5'8"	132–141	138–152	147–166
5'9"	136–145	142–156	151–170
5'10"	140–150	146–160	155–174
5'11"	144–154	150–165	159–179
6'0"	148–158	154–170	164–184
6'1"	152–162	158–175	168–189
6'2"	156–167	162–180	173–194
6'3"	160–171	167–185	178–199
6'4"	164–175	172–190	182–204

Average Weights for Women 25 and Over
(for women between 18 and 25, subtract 1 pound for each year under 25)

HEIGHT (SHOES ON 2″ HEELS)	SMALL FRAME	MEDIUM FRAME	LARGE FRAME
4′10″	92– 98	96–107	104–119
4′11″	94–101	98–110	106–122
5′0″	96–104	101–113	109–125
5′1″	99–107	104–116	112–128
5′2″	102–110	107–119	115–131
5′3″	105–113	110–122	118–134
5′4″	108–116	113–126	121–138
5′5″	111–119	116–130	125–142
5′6″	114–123	120–135	129–146
5′7″	118–127	124–139	133–150
5′8″	122–131	128–143	137–154
5′9″	126–135	132–147	141–158
5′10″	130–140	136–151	145–163
5′11″	134–144	140–155	149–168
6′0″	138–148	144–159	153–173

* From Metropolitan Life Insurance statistics.

to twenty, or even thirty, pounds that many of us are carrying is detrimental to our *physical* health. As clearly delineated by one of the leading authorities about risks and obesity, Dr. Ancel Keys, we have been misled into thinking that minimal obesity or, more accurately, overweight, is a health hazard.

Dr. Keys pointed out that the first source of confusion relates to what we have been using as our standard for "normal" or "ideal" or "desirable" weight: the Metropolitan Life Insurance Table of Average Weights for Men and Women, as shown in Table 12. According to this table, the top "desirable" weight for a 6-foot man of medium frame is 170 pounds. According to the body mass index shown in Figure 14, that weight is well below the 30 figure that is associated with increased risk for cardiovascular disease.

The discrepancy results from the basis for the widely used Metropolitan Table: the weights are based on a group of applicants for life insurance who were in their mid-twenties. These applicants obviously were not representative of the entire normal population and certainly shouldn't be used as the standard for people in their forties, fifties, and sixties. Another source of confusion has been attacked by Dr. Keys: the division into "small," "medium," and "large" frames. He points out that these presumed frame sizes were never measured and were simply created to handle the rather wide range in weights seen among healthy people in their mid-twenties.

In fact, the average weight of American men aged 40 to 59 years is about 15 percent above the "desirable" weight figure for men of "average frame." The question then arises—are the majority of us at an increased risk?

Here again, Dr. Keys is concise and decisive, his views based upon his interpretation of a large body of information. He states that "The idea has been greatly oversold that the risk of dying prematurely or of having a heart attack is directly related to the relative body weight. For middle-aged men, the best prospect for avoiding death in 10 or 15 years is to be about average, or a bit over, in relative weight. The risk rises somewhat with departure in either direction from the happy middle ground, but risk increases substantially only at the extremes of under- and overweight."[1]

The information now available isn't adequate to say much about younger men or women, though they seem to be like the middle-aged men, with no evidence of increased risk for the majority whose weights are average or slightly higher. Remember that these "average" weights are about 15 percent higher than the "desirable" weights listed in the Metropolitan Table.

Another point needs to be emphasized: there are also greater risks for those who are 15 to 20 percent *below* average weight. Though it used to be said that "one could never be too rich or too thin," the truth is that too thin is harmful. This has been shown clearly in the Framingham study. There, death rates were definitely higher in men and women whose relative weight was 10 percent or more below the average. Thus, the curve for weight as it relates to coronary death rates is not a straight line that goes progressively up with increasing weight. Rather, it is a gently sloping U-curve, with increasing trouble for those who are too thin (more than 10 percent below average) and those who are too fat (more than 20 percent above average) (Figure 15).

Even if they do not have physical dysfunction or greater mortality, those who are minimally overweight do carry a handicap. Their problem has been nicely stated by Dr. Faith T. Fitzgerald:

> It is clear from reading magazines or watching television that public derision and condemnation of fat people is one of the few remaining sanctioned prejudices in this nation freely allowed against any group based solely on appearance. Personality profiles of obese adolescent girls show that they respond very much like oppressed minorities in their acceptance of dominant values in the culture and their passive withdrawal. It has been documented that all of us—the general public, social workers, employers, graduate schools admissions officers, nurses and physicians—feel negatively toward the obese. Obesity is a moral crime and one of the few remaining sinful diseases: one is fat because of weakness of the will. The fat are denied jobs, promotions, educational opportunities and, recently, challenged in their right to adopt a child until they lose weight.[2]

This public perception of the obese as "sinful" and "weak" is obviously shared by most who are overweight. This cannot help but be a major psychological trauma and may, in fact, be responsible for much of the frustration that causes them to continue to overeat. They then enter the vicious cycle of increased food intake→obesity→increased food intake→greater

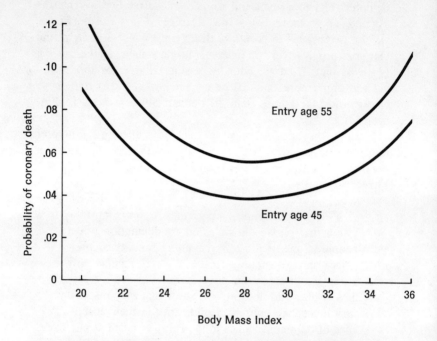

Figure 15. The U-shaped curve relating initial body mass index as a measure of weight to the probability of death from coronary heart disease among 45- and 55-year-old men employed by the Chicago Gas Company who were followed for 14 years. (Source: Keys, A., *Nutrition Reviews* 38 [1980]: 297)

obesity. Most psychologists find no evidence of abnormal emotional patterns before obesity develops. Once people are obese, however, problems do arise.

You cannot look at television or read a magazine without recognizing that our "ideal" female body image is one of extreme thinness, with flat chests and prominent cheekbones, an appearance that is almost emaciated. Not too long ago, things were a great deal different (Figure 16). The models

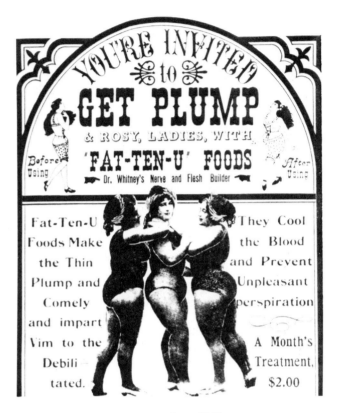

Figure 16. An advertisement from 1910.

of 1900 were, at the least, pleasingly plump. One can't be sure about the reasons for this change in popular perceptions; but whatever the reason, the fat suffer.

This suffering can take some weird turns. We've known that some people—almost all of them young white women—develop a serious physical and psychological aversion to food called *anorexia nervosa*. Even more common, perhaps, may be a pattern alternating between gorging and purging, which has been called *bulimia nervosa*. "Pigging out" is followed by fasting, induced vomiting, or purging with laxatives.

This isn't to say that most fat people enjoy such abuse either self-directed or imposed by society. Teacher Suzanne Jordan, who described herself as "stately and plump" in a *Newsweek* essay, wrote: "Some people say the business about the jolly fat person is a myth, that all of us chubbies are neurotic, sick, sad people. I disagree. Fat people may not be chortling all day long, but they're a hell of a lot nicer than the wizened and shriveled. Thin people turn surly, mean and hard at a younger age because they never learn the value of a hot-fudge sundae for easing tension. Thin people don't like gooey soft things because they themselves are neither gooey nor soft. They are crunchy and dull, like carrots."[3]

THE CAUSES OF OBESITY

As you probably already know, it's tough to lose excess weight. So let us examine what is known about the causes of obesity, with hopes of uncovering some ways to prevent the problem. Regardless of what we find, there are only two ways weight can be gained—either too many calories are taken in or too few calories are burned. No living creature has been known to disobey the basic laws of thermodynamics.

Too Many Calories Coming In

Ordinarily we keep our body weight rather remarkably constant, varying only a few ounces from week to week or year to year. This has given rise to the idea that we have a *ponderostat* or *appestat,* a device that regulates appetite like a thermostat, causing us to eat until a certain amount of body fat is present and then shutting off the appetite. A few people become fat after brain damage that affects an area, the hypothalamus, where appetite seems to be controlled. But for most who are obese, there is no evidence of an abnormality in such an area. It is true most of us cut down on our food intake if given a high-calorie snack before a meal, while some fat people go ahead and eat just as much. Similarly, when lean men were purposely stuffed for long periods, their weights rose a certain amount but when they quit stuffing, their weights fell back to their initial level.[4]

There may, however, be a time when overfeeding leads to permanent obesity. This was first demonstrated in experiments on rodents by Drs. Jules Hirsch, Jerome Knittle, and coworkers at the Rockefeller University. They took groups of newborn rats who were littermates and therefore genetically similar and placed half of these in groups of four to a nursing mother, the other half of them in groups of twenty-two to one mother. Those in the overfed first group not only gained more weight while being nursed but continued to become fatter after weaning as well. When the experimenters counted the number of fat cells in the two groups of rats, they found three times more in those overfed as infants, despite the fact that they must have started life with the same number as their underfed brothers and sisters.

After this report, studies on humans showed the same phenomenon: children or adults with lifelong obesity have increased numbers of fat cells.[5] Those who become obese in adult life tend only to have larger fat cells but no increase in their number. The critical times for developing increased numbers of fat cells by overfeeding seem to be the first year of life and then again around age 10. Presumably, once these fat cells appear, they never disappear, so the person is more likely to gain weight and to have trouble in losing it.

Not all fat babies turn into fat adults and most fat adults were not fat babies. But keeping babies from getting fat seems eminently sensible: it may prevent some of our lifelong troubles.

Fat parents could have fat babies because they overfeed them from infancy on. But another possibility is that fat parents also may be passing on genes which cause their children to become obese. Other than for a few, very rare diseases, there really is no evidence for a genetic inheritance. A shared environment is the likely cause of similar weight patterns seen among family members.

A number of fascinating studies have investigated what turns appetite off and on in nonobese and obese people. As an example, a few people in each category were brought into a hospital where they obtained all of their food, and as much as they wanted, by sucking a liquid concoction out of a container—certainly an unappetizing way to eat. The nonobese subjects, despite the situation, continued to consume about the same number of calories. But the obese people, despite having started at a higher level of caloric intake, immediately cut their consumption. When the circumstances were unattractive, they reduced their caloric intake markedly.[6]

This study, along with a number of others, suggests that obese people often eat in response to external circumstances rather than from internal stimuli. When the surroundings are attractive, they eat even if not driven by some hunger sensation. When the external cues—a cozy place, friends and family around, the TV set on—are gone, they reduce their eating. For many, particularly the poor and unattractive, eating is one of the few gratifications available—and so the cycle continues: more eating→ increased obesity→more eating.

Too Few Calories Going Out

Although those who are markedly overweight almost certainly overeat, the cause of much of our middle-age spread is a decreased expenditure of calories. As we grow older, we slow down in various ways—less dancing, less walking, more sitting behind a desk as a junior executive rather than pounding the pavement as a salesman.

Such subtle differences in physical activity may be responsible for more obesity than we assume. The amount of walking done in a week's time by groups of obese women was compared to that done by a group of normal-weight women, whose life situations (size of home, number of children, and so on) were similar. In one week's time, the normal-weight women walked 34 miles. In the same time, while doing apparently the same amount of housework, shopping, and other tasks, the obese women walked an average of 14 miles.[7] If a mile of walking is worth 100 calories, the obese women would have burned 2,000 fewer calories, enough for more than one-half pound of fat.

That's more than 25 pounds in a year, far more than most gain even under the worst circumstances.

In another study, a series of photographs was taken to measure the times that groups of girls playing tennis were physically active, running around the court, jumping, and burning calories. The group of obese girls was inactive for much longer periods while playing than was the group of nonobese girls.[8]

It is certainly possible that these obese people were less physically active *because* they were obese—it takes more energy to move when you're carrying an extra fifty pounds. So the lesser physical activity may have been the result and not the primary cause of the obesity. Regardless, it certainly worsened the situation.

It may be that those of us who are more efficient, who waste fewer calories in meaningless movement and motion, are more likely to become obese. The obese may not just be outwardly more efficient; they may also have more efficient metabolic machinery within their bodies, burning fewer calories to keep warm, to exercise, and to run the heart, lungs, and other body processes. There are some bits of evidence suggesting various differences in the metabolic efficiency of the obese but, taken together, they are rather unconvincing.

One obvious difference may be involved: many calories are burned to make heat to keep our body temperature at 98°F when the environment is 72°F or colder. Fat is a great insulator—witness the larger amount of body fat in Eskimos—and as more fat is deposited, we need to burn fewer calories to keep our temperatures higher than the outside.

THE TREATMENT OF OBESITY

For most persons wanting to lose weight the problems of both calorie intake and calorie expenditure must be attacked. The verb *attacked* came to me quite naturally. But an "attack" upon your obesity is not what we're really after. That connotes a massive force that is used to achieve a goal in as short a time as possible. It sounds like what most of us have been doing—is it Atkins, Stillman, grapefruit, Mayo, or Beverly Hills this season? Every four to six months, another attack is announced by the publication of another fad diet, sure to become number one on the *New York Times* bestseller list and gain the author appearances on a dozen TV talk shows.

Every one of these attacks works—for about four weeks. The enemy, however, hardly notices, and soon all the weight that was lost is regained; often a bit more is added. After all, every time you fall for one of the fads and fail—as you almost certainly will—you've put your already fragile ego through another roller-coaster ride to nowhere. Failure means more frustration, which only naturally leads to more eating.

So, let's try to be more sensible, planning a "gentle seduction" rather than a "massive attack." The following guidelines should give you an idea of what we're after.

Guidelines for Successful Weight Loss

1. Set sensible short-term goals for yourself. If you're 75 pounds overweight, the idea of shedding all of that in a short period of time is so overwhelming that most people give up in desperation. Go after 5 or 10 pounds at a time and feel good when you've managed that.

2. Recognize that the tendency to be overweight is an incurable but controllable condition, in many ways like hypertension. You've got to establish a new set of eating habits.

3. Go slowly and be thankful for small blessings. It doesn't seem like you're accomplishing much if you lose 1 pound a week, but remember that's 52 pounds in a year! Since it took you 5 or maybe 10 years to gain that much, try to accept a gradual but steady weight loss as a reasonable goal.

4. Weigh in only once a week so as not to

become frustrated by a slow weight loss. If you accomplish your short-term goal, reward yourself with a nonfattening treat. You may want to go on a "maintenance" diet for a few weeks before taking off another 5 to 10 pounds, or you may be so flushed by victory as to want to go right on.

5. Use some techniques to modify your eating behavior: prepare only enough food for the meal; put the food on the plate (a small one) without having extra portions at the table; eat without distractions, never in front of the TV set; eat slowly; realize that it is not a sin to leave food on your plate; the starving will not find out.

6. If your willpower fails and you give in to temptation, try to be satisfied with the first few bites of "forbidden" foods. And when you do give in, recognize that you're only human. Falling off the wagon temporarily needn't mean that you have to lose the whole wagon and the horse as well.

7. Eat 3 meals a day and always have low-calorie snacks available. You never know when the urge will strike and you must be ready with carrots, cauliflower, or other ammunition.

8. Don't look for magic from pills or spas. They may provide temporary help, but it still gets down to cutting calories—roughly 500 a day below what you burn in order to lose a pound a week since there are 3,500 calories in a pound of fat.

9. Exercise as much as you can, starting slowly and gradually building up your capacity. Be sensible about the form of exercise you perform. Few people will stick with jogging a mile every day. But everyone can walk an

extra mile a day, particularly if it's 6 blocks to the office or shopping center. Make this part of your regular routine and not a time-consuming extra effort that quickly becomes such a burden that you quit. A mile of brisk walking a day burns about 90 calories, enough to shed 7 pounds in a year (see Table 13, "Calories Expended in Various Activities").

10. Remember that beer and booze have lots of calories (see Table 14, "Calorie Content of Alcoholic Beverages"). Lower-calorie beer and wine are available but a 6-pack of lite beer is still almost 600 calories.

Special Diet Programs

You may find that Weight Watchers or the less expensive TOPS groups are your easiest way to successful weight loss. Their ideas and diets are sound, but some people get turned off by the public exposure and by some of the gimmicks. However, being involved with other people who are struggling with you—and being guided by people who have been successful—should help.

In the last few years, a number of more stringent diet programs have been established with physicians, psychologists, and nutritionists involved. One of the most popular, introduced by Dr. Victor Vertes in Cleveland, uses five packets a day containing a total of 45 grams of protein along with some minerals and vitamins and providing 300 calories. Initially, no food is eaten and weight loss has often been greater than the expected two pounds per week.[9] As with all very low-calorie diets, much of the initial weight loss is fluid and not fat. According to this plan, the "modified fast with supplemental protein" is supplemented with food after the major amount of weight is lost and the dieter is given an intensive program in behavioral modification.

This program is now available in special obesity clinics in

Table 13: Calories Expended in Various Activities

Activity	Calories per minute
MODERATE ACTIVITY	
Bicycling (5½ mph)	3.5
Walking (2½ mph)	3.5
Gardening	3.6
Canoeing (2½ mph)	3.8
Golf	4.2
Bowling	4.5
Lawn mowing (hand mower)	4.5
Fencing	5.0
Swimming (¼ mph)	5.0
Walking (3¾ mph)	5.0
Badminton, volleyball	6.0
Horseback riding (trotting)	6.0
Roller skating	6.0
Square dancing	6.0
VIGOROUS ACTIVITY	
Ice skating (10 mph)	7.0
Tennis	7.0
Hill climbing (100 ft. per hr)	8.0
Water skiing	8.0
Skiing (10 mph)	10.0
Squash and handball	10.0
Cycling (13 mph)	11.0
Running (10 mph)	15.0

many large cities, and a similar low-calorie diet powder is widely sold as "the Cambridge Diet." It appears to be safe and, according to initial reports, quite effective. However, similar claims have been made for other stringent diet programs, including prolonged total starvation. Despite impressive weight loss *during* starvation, almost every subject regained every pound

Table 14: Calorie Content of Alcoholic Beverages

	Size	Calories
SPIRITS		
80 proof: gin, rum, vodka, whiskey, brandy	1½ ounces	105
MIXED DRINKS		
Bloody Mary	3 ounces	80
Manhattan	3 ounces	183
Daiquiri	3 ounces	213
Martini	3 ounces	215
Brandy Alexander	3 ounces	237
Grasshopper	3 ounces	264
Old Fashioned	3 ounces	270
CORDIALS		
Liqueurs	⅔ ounce	66
Brandy, cognac	1 ounce	73
WINES		
Table: 10% alcohol		
Champagne	4 ounces	84
Red and white, dry vermouth	4 ounces	90
Sweet: 15% alcohol		
Port, sherry	2 ounces	84
Wine, sweet vermouth	2 ounces	140
BEER		
Lite (1 can)	12 ounces	96
Regular (1 can)	12 ounces	150
CARBONATED MIXES		
Cola	4 ounces	48
Soda	4 ounces	—

lost when allowed to restart eating. Whether the inclusion of behavioral modification to instill long-term changes in eating habits will make the Vertes program more successful over the long run remains to be proved.

In the meantime, avoid liquid protein diets, since they are associated with a number of deaths due to heart rhythm disturbances. They were the Last Chance Diet in ways certainly not intended by their promoters. Similarly, avoid high fat-low carbohydrate diets (such as Dr. Atkins) since they may raise blood cholesterol levels.

More Conventional Self-Diets

You need to reduce your caloric intake below your caloric expenditure by 500 calories per day to lose 3,500 calories or one pound of fat a week. To lose two pounds of weight per week, a daily deficit of 1,000 calories is needed. That should be accomplished by a combination of decreased intake by a diet and, to a lesser degree, increased expenditure by exercise.

There are many sources of complete diet programs, but you really may not need to do much more than cut out some high-calorie sweets, desserts, breads, and dressings and substitute lower-calorie foods for high-calorie ones, as shown in the listing provided in Table 15 (taken from the booklet "Are You Really Serious about Losing Weight?", supplied by Penwalt Corporation—one of the more sensible programs I've seen).

For more information, consult these books:

> *American Heart Association Cookbook,* David
> McKay, 1979.
> *Living Better: Recipes for a Healthy Heart,* by
> J. D. Margie, R. I. Levy, and J. C. Hunt,
> HLS Press, 1981.
> *Nutrition Scoreboard,* by M. F. Jacobson, Avon,
> 1975.

In addition, a more structured program of behavior modification may prove more helpful than the rather loose one

Table 15: Lower-Calorie Foods to Substitute*

FOR THIS	Calories	SUBSTITUTE THIS	Calories	Calories saved
Beverages				
☐ Milk (whole), 8 oz.	165	Milk (buttermilk, skim) 8 oz.	80	85
☐ Prune juice, 8 oz.	170	Tomato juice, 8 oz.	50	120
☐ Soft drinks, 8 oz.	105	Diet soft drinks, 8 oz.	1	104
☐ Coffee (with cream and 2 tsp. sugar)	110	Coffee (black with artificial sweetener)	0	110
☐ Cocoa (all milk), 8 oz.	235	Cocoa (milk and water), 8 oz.	140	95
☐ Chocolate malted milk shake, 8 oz.	500	Lemonade (sweetened), 8 oz.	100	400
☐ Beer (1 bottle), 12 oz.	175	Liquor (1½ oz.), with soda or water, 8 oz.	120	55
Breakfast foods				
☐ Rice flakes, 1 cup	110	Puffed rice, 1 cup	50	60
☐ Eggs (scrambled), 2	220	Eggs (boiled, poached), 2	160	60
Butter and Cheese				
☐ Butter on toast	170	Apple butter on toast	90	80
☐ Cheese (Blue, Cheddar, Cream, Swiss), 1 oz.	105	Cheese (cottage, uncreamed), 1 oz.	25	80
Desserts				
☐ Angel food cake, 2″ piece	110	Cantaloupe melon, ½	40	70
☐ Cheese cake, 2″ piece	200	Watermelon, ½″ slice (10″ diam.)	60	140
☐ Chocolate cake with icing, 2″ piece	425	Sponge cake, 2″ piece	120	305
☐ Fruit cake, 2″ piece	115	Grapes, 1 cup	65	50
☐ Pound cake, 1 oz. piece	140	Plums, 2	50	90
☐ Cupcake, white icing, 1	230	Plain cupcake, 1	115	115

* From "Are You Really Serious about Losing Weight?", 14th edition. Rochester, N.Y.: Penwalt Corp., 1981, pp. 46–49.

Table 15—Continued

FOR THIS	Calories	SUBSTITUTE THIS	Calories	Calories saved
☐ Cookies, assorted (3″ diam.), 1	120	Vanilla wafer (dietetic), 1	25	95
☐ Ice cream, 4 oz.	150	Yogurt (flavored), 4 oz.	60	90
Pie				
☐ Apple, 1 piece (⅐ of a 9″ pie)	345	Tangerine (fresh), 1	40	305
☐ Blueberry, 1 piece	290	Blueberries (frozen, unsweetened), ½ cup	45	245
☐ Cherry, 1 piece	355	Cherries (whole), ½ cup	40	315
☐ Custard, 1 piece	280	Banana, small, 1	85	195
☐ Lemon meringue, 1 piece	305	Lemon-flavored gelatin, ½ cup	70	235
☐ Peach,1 piece	280	Peach (whole), 1	35	245
☐ Rhubarb,1 piece	265	Grapefruit, ½	55	210
☐ Pudding (flavored), ½ cup	140	Pudding (dietetic, nonfat milk), ½ cup	60	80
Fish and Fowl				
☐ Tuna (canned), 3 oz.	165	Crabmeat (canned), 3 oz.	80	85
☐ Oysters (fried), 6	400	Oysters (shell w/sauce), 6	100	300
☐ Ocean perch (fried), 4 oz.	260	Bass, 4 oz.	105	155
☐ Fish sticks, 5 sticks or 4 oz.	200	Swordfish (broiled), 3 oz.	140	60
☐ Lobster meat, 4 oz. with 2 tbsp. butter	300	Lobster meat, 4 oz., with lemon	95	205
☐ Duck (roasted), 3 oz.	310	Chicken (roasted), 3 oz.	160	150

Table 15—Continued

FOR THIS   SUBSTITUTE THIS

Meats	Calo-ries		Calo-ries	Calo-ries saved
☐ Loin roast, 3 oz.	290	Pot roast (round), 3 oz.	160	130
☐ Rump roast, 3 oz.	290	Rib roast, 3 oz.	200	90
☐ Swiss steak, 3½ oz.	300	Liver (fried), 2½ oz.	210	90
☐ Hamburger (av. fat, broiled), 3 oz.	240	Hamburger (lean, broiled), 3 oz.	145	95
☐ Porterhouse steak, 3 oz.	250	Club steak, 3 oz.	160	90
☐ Rib lamb chop (med.), 3 oz.	300	Lamb leg roast (lean only), 3 oz.	160	140
☐ Pork chop (med.), 3 oz.	340	Veal chop (med.), 3 oz.	185	155
☐ Pork roast, 3 oz.	310	Veal roast, 3 oz.	230	80
☐ Pork sausage, 3 oz.	405	Ham (boiled, lean), 3 oz.	200	205
Potatoes				
☐ Fried, 1 cup	480	Baked (2½" diam.)	100	380
☐ Mashed, 1 cup	245	Boiled (2½" diam.)	100	145
Salads				
☐ Chef salad with oil dressing, 1 tbsp.	180	Chef salad with dietetic dressing, 1 tbsp.	40	140
☐ Chef salad with mayonnaise, 1 tbsp.	125	Chef salad with dietetic dressing, 1 tbsp.	40	85
☐ Chef salad with Roquefort, Blue, Russian, French dressing 1 tbsp.	105	Chef salad with dietetic dressing, 1 tbsp.	40	65
Sandwiches				
☐ Club	375	Bacon and tomato (open)	200	175

Table 15—Continued

FOR THIS	Calories	SUBSTITUTE THIS	Calories	Calories saved
☐ Peanut butter and jelly	275	Egg salad (open)	165	110
☐ Turkey with gravy, 3 tbsp.	520	Hamburger, lean (open), 3 oz.	200	320
Snacks				
☐ Fudge, 1 oz.	115	Vanilla wafers (dietetic) 2	50	65
☐ Peanuts (salted), 1 oz.	170	Apple, 1	100	70
☐ Peanuts (roasted), 1 cup, shelled	1375	Grapes, 1 cup	65	1310
☐ Potato chips, 10 med.	115	Pretzels, 10 small sticks	35	80
☐ Chocolate, 1 oz. bar	145	Toasted marshmallows, 3	75	70
Soups				
☐ Creamed, 1 cup	210	Chicken noodle, 1 cup	110	100
☐ Bean, 1 cup	190	Beef noodle, 1 cup	110	80
☐ Minestrone, 1 cup	105	Beef bouillon, 1 cup	10	95
Vegetables				
☐ Baked beans, 1 cup	320	Green beans, 1 cup	30	290
☐ Lima beans, 1 cup	160	Asparagus, 1 cup	30	130
☐ Corn (canned), 1 cup	185	Cauliflower, 1 cup	30	155
☐ Peas (canned), 1 cup	145	Peas (fresh), 1 cup	115	30
☐ Winter squash, 1 cup	75	Summer squash, 1 cup	30	45
☐ Succotash, 1 cup	260	Spinach, 1 cup	40	220

described here. When such a program was carefully compared with standard medical practice (monthly office visits, instructions on diet and exercise) and with rather intensive drug therapy for six months, the behavior therapy produced less weight loss during the six-month study, but those who had had the behavior therapy regained much less weight over the ensuing twelve months.[10] In this study, the behavior therapy was the highly structured one described by Ferguson and the Mahoneys. If you want to use such therapy, a group approach working with a psychologist may be best. Sources for more details include:

> *Learning to Eat: Leaders' Manual and Patients' Manual,* by J. M. Ferguson, Bull Publishing Co., 1975.
> *Permanent Weight Control,* by M. H. Mahoney and K. Mahoney, W. W. Norton, 1976.
> *Slim Chance in a Fat World: Behavioral Control of Obesity,* by R. B. Stuart and B. Davis, Research Press, 1972.

When All Else Fails

Drastic measures are sometimes needed for morbid obesity. Persistent use of one or another of the special diet programs should always be attempted first. But if they too fail, surgery may prove lifesaving. Three procedures are currently being done: a jejunoileal bypass, a gastric bypass, and gastroplasty. The first-named procedure has largely been supplanted by one of the gastric procedures. Though weight loss may be excellent, the procedures are dangerous in very fat people and bothersome side effects are frequent. Once again, long-term success may be less than initial results seem to indicate.

Obesity is common and we've not been very successful up to this point in overcoming it. Despite spending well over 10 billion dollars a year on weight-losing methods and ideas, millions of Americans continue on their seemingly hopeless quest for a size 6 figure or a 34-inch waist.

Much more likely to succeed is a program of prevention. Infant feeding habits can be altered to provide adequate nutrition without increasing the child's risks for later obesity or hypertension. The renewed interest in breast-feeding is a good sign. In Stanford, California, children in the fourth and fifth grades of school were given an effective instructional program and altered their own eating behavior, increased their level of physical activity, and influenced their family's eating patterns as well.[11] If we can reach parents and children early enough, healthy eating habits should be easy to adopt and easier to maintain.

SEVEN

Diabetes and Glucose Intolerance

Diabetes is a problem less common than those discussed in preceding chapters. However, for those who have it, diabetes poses a considerable risk for cardiovascular disease. Diabetes develops in about 2 percent of the population and another 2 to 4 percent are considered to be borderline diabetics. Those who have diabetes develop more vascular disease at an earlier age, a process that, until recently, has not been preventable.

A much larger group of people—and this probably includes you, particularly if you are overweight—have a reduced ability to clear the blood of sugar (glucose) after a large load is given in the form of a glucose tolerance test. The finding of glucose intolerance, or a higher blood sugar level, during the two hours after drinking a large quantity of glucose had been thought to pose the danger of premature vascular disease. The evidence for this anticipated increased danger has now been more carefully examined and the danger may have been grossly overstated.

THE RISKS OF DIABETES

Diabetes mellitus is a disease wherein the amount of insulin is inadequate to burn the glucose in the blood so that the level of blood glucose is high even after an overnight fast (a situation called fasting hyperglycemia). Insulin is a hormone produced in the pancreas, a gland sitting in the cradle of the intestines. Insulin enables glucose to enter the cells wherein it can be burned. The energy derived from the metabolism of glucose is used to run various body processes and is essential for normal health.

Diabetes is now classified into two types: Type I is "insulin dependent," requiring that additional insulin be supplied to the patient since there is too little made by the patient's pancreas to sustain life. Type II is "insulin independent," wherein the patient has a deficiency of insulin action but still makes the hormone and does not require additional insulin. There are typically a number of differences between the two types (Table 16).

The smaller group who have Type I diabetes must take daily injections of insulin. In the past, despite these injections, their blood sugar levels were often too high (hyperglycemia) and sometimes too low (hypoglycemia). Their variable blood sugar levels reflect the inability of one, two, or even four shots of insulin to mimic what goes on in the normal body—whenever

Table 16: The Two Types of Diabetes

	Type I	Type II
Need for insulin	Yes	No
Other names	Juvenile-onset, brittle	Adult-onset, stable
Usual age of onset	Before 40	After 40
Association with obesity	Infrequent	Usual
Propensity to acute reactions, ketosis, coma	Marked	Minimal
Response to oral hypoglycemia drugs	None	Usual

119

the blood sugar goes up (with meals and snacks, during times of stress) the pancreas very quickly produces just the amount of insulin needed to use the extra blood sugar. This precise, accurate, and fast response is one of a number of remarkable servomechanisms which control body processes. The Type I diabetic, unable to make any or only very small amounts of insulin, must depend on insulin extracted from animal pancreas glands. This insulin, given as multiple injections, doesn't just come out "on demand." Therefore the diabetic is susceptible to having too high a blood sugar after meals and too low a blood sugar between meals.

A number of other body constituents and processes interact with the blood sugar. When the level of blood sugar fluctuates, these other constituents also go astray. One of the constituents that usually rises is blood cholesterol, and the Type I diabetic usually has a high total cholesterol with a high LDL and a low HDL component, just the pattern described in Chapter 5 known to be associated with the development of atherosclerosis.

With the more common Type II diabetes, insulin can be made by the patient's pancreas but not in adequate amounts to control glucose metabolism. Most Type II diabetics are obese. The presence of increased amounts of body fat and the excessive intake of calories lead to a progressive weakening of the action of insulin. As a result, even though high levels of insulin may be present in the blood, the blood sugar level rises and, along with it, the blood cholesterol level as well.

Type II diabetics usually don't need additional insulin but they may require oral drugs that stimulate their pancreas to make even more of their own insulin and thereby overcome the relative resistance to its actions. A diet with fewer calories so that weight begins to go down is usually much more effective in controlling Type II diabetes than these drugs and even more effective than additional insulin injections.

The diabetic, whether Type I or Type II, is likely to develop vascular disease. This tends to involve the larger blood vessels (macrovascular) such as in the heart and brain, leading to more frequent heart attacks and strokes. In addition, the diabetic suffers from narrowing of and damage to small blood vessels (microvascular) particularly in the eye, kidneys, and skin. As a result, progressive loss of vision, kidney damage, and poor circulation frequently develop in those with long-standing diabetes.

The larger-vessel disease is probably of the same type as that seen in nondiabetics and may be more common in diabetics mainly because they have more of the various risk factors, particularly high cholesterol and obesity. But the smaller-vessel disease may be genetically predetermined, along with the tendency to develop diabetes. Though not all agree, most diabetes experts believe that much of the diabetic's vascular trouble is part of the inherited background of the disease and not a reflection of elevated blood sugar, blood cholesterol, or any other acquired problem.

This genetic connection has dampened the enthusiasm of some physicians and patients, since it promises vascular trouble after a period of years, regardless of what is done about the blood sugar and the rest of the patient's body processes. However, until recently, there really has been no practical way to keep the blood sugar normal enough over a long enough time to really know if the abnormally fluctuating blood sugar—and symptoms that accompany it—is responsible for the trouble.

In the last few years, pumps have been made that can deliver minuscule amounts of insulin continuously and with occasional bursts—closely mimicking the workings of the normal pancreas. Though such insulin pumps, worn on a belt and attached to a needle under the skin over the abdomen, must still be carefully monitored and can only be used in a small number of diabetics, the possibility they provide of virtually normalizing the blood sugar for long periods offers the potential of deciding the issue: is it the abnormal blood sugar or is it an inherited vascular problem which is responsible for the more rapid damage to the diabetic's heart and blood vessels? Reports such as that by Dr. James Falko and associates have already shown that the use of the insulin pump can improve the diabetic's blood lipid status, lowering the LDL cholesterol and raising the HDL cholesterol.[1]

In the not-too-distant future, even better ways of delivering "insulin on demand" will likely be available, possibly along with transplants of pancreas tissue so that the patient can really then do it himself. But for now, we should do what we can: try to control the diabetes carefully; use a diet low in fat and calories to maintain a normal weight and cholesterol level; avoid cigarette smoking; treat hypertension vigorously; and relieve whatever other risks may be present.

ABNORMAL GLUCOSE TOLERANCE

The plight of the diabetic is of serious concern, but there is certainly hope that we can do better. In the meantime, many more of us are thought to be a higher risk because of a lessened ability to clear the blood of glucose after an oral load has been consumed even though our fasting blood sugar levels are perfectly normal. A test for glucose tolerance has been used by physicians for many years as part of the health profile. The Framingham study used such an oral glucose tolerance test (OGTT) as part of the examination and found that those who had either a high fasting blood sugar or an abnormal glucose tolerance test definitely had an increased likelihood of developing cardiovascular disease, twofold higher for men, threefold for women.[2]

No one would dispute that the higher incidence of cardiovascular disease among definite diabetics is a correct finding. But many would argue that those with only abnormal glucose tolerance should not be lumped with the diabetics since most studies limited to the former group have failed to show increased likelihood of vascular disease. Fifteen separate studies involving many thousands of men aged 50 to 59 who were monitored for ten years or longer have been carefully analyzed, with the conclusion that an increased risk was not demonstrated when the other known risk factors were factored out. That is, those with an abnormal glucose tolerance test also tended to be obese, hypertensive, physically inactive, and so on (for other factors associated with glucose intolerance, see Table 17). When these known risk factors were excluded, an

Table 17: Some Factors Associated with Glucose Intolerance

Early diabetes	Liver disease
Pregnancy	Steroid therapy
Obesity	Intestinal disorders
Acute illness	Old age

abnormal glucose tolerance test was not strongly indicative of future trouble.

This may sound irrelevant to you, but a great deal of time and trouble continue to be taken in determining glucose tolerance and worrying about abnormal tolerance. Physicians naturally want to identify everything that is predictive of future trouble. Some may disagree with my position that these tests are really not worth doing.

For now, I advise that you do whatever you can to reduce those factors that may worsen your glucose tolerance. If you have diabetics in your family, be even more careful. But if you are not diabetic, don't be too concerned about an abnormal glucose tolerance.

EIGHT

Physical Activity

Most likely you are one of the 70 million Americans—half of the adult population—who are doing some type of physical exercise on a regular basis, spending over $30 billion a year in the process. Your reasons for exercising probably include the belief that you are improving your cardiovascular fitness and, thereby, reducing your chance for heart disease. You may be right but, despite all those hours of jogging and millions of pushups, we really aren't certain about the benefits of physical exercise for the majority of us.

Part of the problem in determining what exercise does for our heart health is our inability to examine the effect of exercise by itself. If you become a regular jogger, you will probably also change your diet, lose weight, quit smoking, reduce your drinking, and who knows what else. If good things happen as a result—as they probably will—how can we be sure they happened as a result of jogging?

Some will say, "Who cares? If all these changes occur because you start to jog, give jogging the credit." But we do need to know, first because jogging and other forms of exercise do have costs and potential hazards; second, because if they work, we need to know why and then we need to get everyone involved.

Though hardly a new activity in human experience, exercise has literally taken off just in the past ten years. Much is being learned about its potential benefits but a great deal more needs to be learned.

THE RISKS OF PHYSICAL INACTIVITY

We will look further at what is known about the potential positive effects of exercise but let's start by seeing what is known about the possible negative effects of physical inactivity.

A number of studies have looked at both the occurrence of and death rates from coronary artery disease in relation to the level of physical activity at work and during leisure time. They have involved groups (mostly men) as diverse as London bus drivers, San Francisco longshoremen, and Harvard graduates. Though a few have not, most have shown a definite relation: the more physical activity, the less heart disease.

One of the larger and longer studies is by Dr. R. S. Paffenbarger, Jr., and associates involving almost four thousand San Francisco longshoremen who were monitored for twenty-two years. When their level of work activity, graded from 1 (the lowest) to 7 (the highest), was related to their relative risk for having a fatal heart attack, the risk was found to go down progressively, the harder the work and the younger the men (Figure 17).

Greater physical activity during leisure time has also been shown to be associated with less death and disability from heart disease. Almost eighteen hundred British civil servants were divided into two groups by Dr. J. N. Morris and colleagues and monitored from 1968 to 1970: the group that engaged in vigorous exercise had less than half of the number of deaths and cases of coronary heart disease than the group that did not.[1] Vigorous exercise was defined as strenuous sports or heavy work around the house on the weekend before the interview.

In both these studies, the differences in rates of heart disease could not be attributed to differences in other risk factors

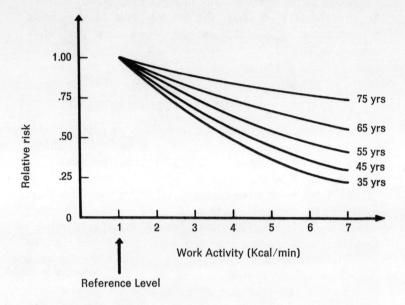

Figure 17. The estimated relative risk of fatal heart attack is shown to fall progressively with increasing levels of work activity for men at various ages, based upon the experience among San Francisco longshoremen followed over a 22-year period. (Source: Brand, R. J.; Paffenbarger, R. S., Jr.; Sholtz, R. I.; and Kampert, J. B., "Work Activity and Fatal Heart Attack Studied by Multiple Logistic Risk Analysis," *American Journal of Epidemiology* 110 [1979]: 53)

(such as smoking and hypertension) between the different groups.

As impressive as these studies are, there are problems with using them as proof that increasing physical activity, at work or play, is protective against heart disease. The main problem was clearly shown by analysis of the first major report on the

126

relationship between physical activity and heart disease (published in 1953 by the same Dr. J. N. Morris who later on studied the civil servants). In that 1953 study, physically inactive London bus drivers, who sit all day, were compared with physically active London bus conductors, who are constantly walking and climbing up and down the double-decker buses: the drivers had twice the rate of heart disease. The authors originally warned that this difference could reflect self-selection: the coronary-prone might be more likely to seek easier work as a driver than as a conductor.

Dr. Morris and coworkers looked further at their two groups in 1966. The bus drivers were in fact at higher risk for heart disease for multiple reasons: they were heavier and they had higher serum cholesterol and higher blood pressures than the conductors. So the situation is confounded: the bus drivers may have started off in worse shape or, because of their physical inactivity, they may have become progressively more out of shape. Either way, physical activity cannot, by itself, be given credit for the lower rate of heart disease among the conductors.

There are other problems with such studies. People may work hard but loaf at home or vice versa; they may change their levels of activity after being classified; it may be hard to know just how much activity is involved in different jobs. Remember, there were longshoremen who had very low levels of work activity.

MECHANISMS BY WHICH PHYSICAL ACTIVITY MAY PROTECT YOU

Regardless of these potential pitfalls, a large number of carefully performed studies do show a lesser rate of heart disease among those who are more active at work or at play. The reasons for this are multiple, some related to direct effects on the heart and circulation, others to indirect effects on other risk factors.

First, let us note the important difference between the two major types of physical exercise:

- *isotonic* or *dynamic* or *aerobic* exercise involves rhythmical contractions and relaxations of large muscles, as with walking, running, or swimming.
- *isometric* or *static* exercise involves increased muscular tension against a fixed resistance with no significant movement, as with heavy weight lifting or pushing against a wall.

Some exercises, such as pushups and most Nautilus-type activities, combine both movements to varying degrees, often starting with an isometric push and ending with an isotonic movement.

The term *aerobic* (with air), popularized by Dr. Kenneth Cooper, simply refers to exercise of a mild-to-moderate intensity that uses oxygen to supply the energy for muscle contractions. On the other hand, exercise that is done without air ("anaerobic") uses sources of energy without oxygen. Anaerobic exercises include high-intensity short bursts, such as a 100-yard-dash or heavy weight lifting. As aerobic exercise continues and the supply of oxygen is exhausted, the body turns more and more to anaerobic metabolism. Thereafter, it takes a long time to restore the body's supply of oxygen, as reflected in prolonged breathlessness.

In general, isometric exercise does no good for you except to enlarge your muscles—important really only for football linemen and weight lifters. In fact, during the time the muscles are tightened, a reflex acutely constricts the blood vessels and increases the heart rate, causing the blood pressure to rise markedly (Figure 18). This is potentially harmful and without doubt explains the strokes and heart attacks occasionally seen when strenuous isometric exercise such as shoveling heavy snow or pushing against a stuck window is performed.

The Potential Benefits of Isotonic Exercise

Isotonic exercises, on the other hand, improve cardiovascular fitness, bringing about greater efficiency in the functions of

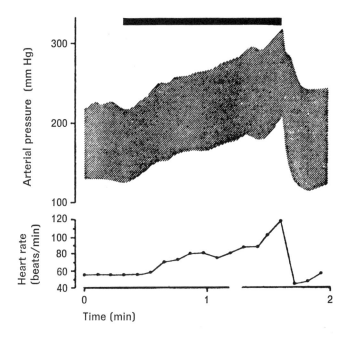

Figure 18. The effect of a one-minute period of isometric exercise (handgrip at 50% of maximum contraction), shown as the black bar, upon the blood pressure and heart rate of a hypertensive patient. (Source: Ewing, D. J. *et al., British Heart Journal* 35 [1973]: 413)

the heart and lungs and improving their ability to withstand sudden stresses. In addition to reducing other risk factors, the ways isotonic exercise may help include these facts:

- The heart pumps more blood and the tissues remove a greater amount of oxygen from the blood, resulting in an increased *maximal oxygen uptake,* the best measure of a person's fitness. This is the factor measured during most "stress tests."

- The heart is able to do more work at a lower heart rate, allowing it to be a more efficient pump.
- The blood supply to the heart muscle increases. This occurrence has been shown in animals but not with certainty in man.
- The heart is less likely to develop life-threatening disturbances in its rhythm when its blood supply is reduced.
- The blood tends not to clot as quickly, reducing the tendency to form obstructive thromboses, the cause of many acute heart attacks.
- The heart may respond less chaotically to acute stresses or unusual effort.

How you can achieve these potential protective effects is discussed below, but let's now see what exercise may do to some of the other known risk factors for cardiovascular disease.

The main advantages of regular isotonic exercise may be to reduce some additional risk factors: obesity, high blood cholesterol, hypertension, glucose intolerance, psychological stress, and the frequency of engaging in other detrimental health habits, such as smoking. Claims have been made that all of these may be reduced by regular exercise. However, a recent report from Australia by Dr. Antony Sedgwick and his colleagues showed some sobering facts: of 370 sedentary men who started a regular exercise program, only one-third were still exercising five years later.[2] But even more disturbing was the lack of improvement in any of the accompanying risk factors among those who did continue exercising. Though they became more physically fit, they achieved no fall in weight, blood pressure, blood cholesterol, or smoking habits. These men did only moderate exercise: one hour of calisthenics, interval running, and volleyball twice a week. Some would argue that wasn't enough, but it was enough to improve their physical fitness by 17 percent (as measured by an exercise stress test) and it is probably more than most of us would do on a regular basis.

Despite this sobering report (and there are at least two others showing similar lack of other good results from exercise), there do seem to be possibilities of helping control the following problems:

- Obesity: Though even vigorous exercise cannot induce rapid weight loss, a regular isotonic exercise program can be an important component of the long-range weight-loss program described in Chapter 6 that is most likely to achieve significant success. A number of variables determine how many calories will be burned during exercise, including:

  1. The amount of muscular activity required: for a 160-pound man to burn 120 calories, he must run 1.6 km (one mile), walk 2.4 km (1.5 miles), or bicycle 4.8 km (3 miles). (Table 13, page 109, describes the calories expended in various activities.)
  2. The weight of the person doing the exercise (see Table 18, "Caloric Values for Running 1.5 Miles"). A 120-pound person running 1.5 miles in 10 minutes burns 121 calories; a 220-pound man running at the same rate burns 219 calories.
  3. On the other hand, the speed of running the distance makes little difference: a 120-pound person running 1.5 miles in eight minutes burns 125 calories; if the time is doubled to 16 minutes, 112 calories are still burned (see Table 19).

- Hypertension: In a follow-up study of a large number of Harvard graduates, R. S. Paffenbarger, Jr., and colleagues found that those who were physically active had less hyperten-

Table 18: Caloric Values for Running 1.5 Miles (2.4 km)

Weight									Minutes to run 1.5 miles			
LB	KG	8	9	10	11	12	13	14	15	16
120	54.5	125	124	121	120	119	117	116	114	112
130	59.0	124	133	132	130	128	126	125	123	121
140	63.6	145	143	141	139	138	136	134	132	130
150	68.1	155	153	151	149	147	145	143	141	139
160	72.6	165	163	161	159	156	154	152	150	148
170	77.2	175	173	170	168	166	164	161	159	157
180	81.7	185	182	180	178	175	173	171	168	166
190	86.3	195	192	190	187	185	182	180	177	175
200	90.8	205	202	199	197	194	192	189	186	184
210	95.3	215	212	209	206	204	201	198	195	193
220	99.9	225	222	219	216	213	210	207	204	202

sion.[3] There have been reports involving small groups of hypertensive people whose blood pressure was reduced by an exercise program.[4] However, as noted in Chapter 4, weight loss is a fairly certain way to lower the blood pressure and it's likely that the effects of exercise are mediated by its associated effect on weight.

· Blood cholesterol: Physically active people tend to have higher levels of the protective HDL cholesterol and a number of studies have shown favorable changes in the blood cholesterol levels in men who exercise moderately to strenuously. These include a decrease in both total and LDL cholesterol as well as an increase in the HDL cholesterol. Similar favorable changes in blood cholesterol levels were shown in a group of monkeys on a high cholesterol diet who were exercised regularly. Most impressively, those who exercised had larger coronary arteries (not unexpected) and much less atherosclerotic narrowing of these arteries (not unexpected but never before shown so clearly—see Figure 19). Whether people can obtain such protection from exercise remains to be seen.

· Glucose tolerance: Improvements in the abnormal glucose tolerance and the resistance to insulin seen with obesity and diabetes have been recorded after a vigorous walking program.

· Psychological effects: Many joggers describe a virtual addiction to their exercise, feeling "high" when they are running and "withdrawal" when they cannot. The body produces a natural opiumlike hormone (endorphin) and its levels have been found to be increased after one-hour periods of high-intensity running, the increases becoming greater after

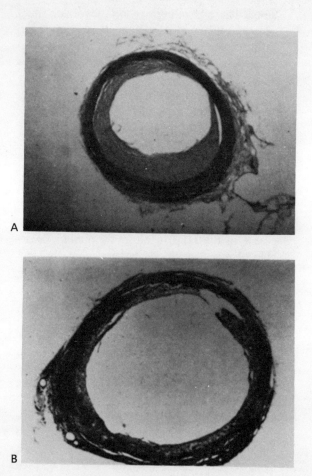

Figure 19. The appearance of the main coronary artery in two monkeys on the same high-fat and cholesterol diet for 24 months. The upper photo (**A**) is of the sedentary monkey, showing 52% narrowing of the lumen by atheroma. The lower photo (**B**) is of the exercise-conditioned monkey, showing only 7% narrowing. In addition, the artery of the exercised monkey is considerably larger. (Source: Kramsch, D. M. *et al., New England Journal of Medicine* 305 [1981]: 1483. Reprinted by permission of the New England Journal of Medicine.)

physical conditioning was accomplished. Even without achieving a "high," many find that exercise provides a good outlet for their tensions while promoting a sense of well-being and a better self-image. As we shall see in the next chapter, people with a Type A behavior-pattern, characterized as being more aggressive and having a heightened sense of time urgency, have more heart disease. After ten weeks of walking and jogging for three miles three times weekly, a group of healthy adults was found to have less of the Type A characteristics. If this change persisted, they presumably would reduce their cardiovascular risk.

THE RISKS OF EXERCISE

All of this sounds great, but remember the Australian study, one of the few carefully controlled and carried out over a long period, which showed absolutely no effect of moderate exercise on any of these risk factors. Though the evidence for benefits from exercise, then, remains equivocal, let's accept the popular belief that it helps.

On the other hand, exercise *can* do harm—if it's overdone by people in poor condition who want to make up for lost time in a hurry. As described by Dr. Robert Eliot, these "weekend warriors" are "drag racing in a used car that has never been checked out." [5] The strain upon the heart of strenuous exercise in an untrained person with previously unrecognized narrowing of the coronary arteries may be enough to cause permanent damage. For that reason, those over age 40 are advised to have a thorough physical exam and perhaps a stress test before beginning a heavy exercise program. On the other hand, if you begin a walking program and slowly increase the distance and speed, there should be little risk. If chest pain, irregular heart beats, undue fatigue, or any peculiar symptoms develop during any form of exercise, the exercise should be stopped and medical attention sought. Rarely, but still too often, sudden death accompanies sudden surges of exercise. And despite a popular misconception, even those who have run a 26-mile marathon can, and do, die of heart disease— though probably a lot fewer do than the rest of us.

A REASONABLE EXERCISE PROGRAM

A regular isotonic exercise program will help you feel and look better—and it may help you live longer. If done correctly, it should cost you little more than some time and a new pair of athletic shoes. However, since its significant benefit to cardiovascular health remains to be proven, don't join the jogging craze with the certain expectation that it will decrease your risk of heart disease and prolong your life. One of my cardiology colleagues once said, "Joggers don't really live longer—it just seems like it."

You don't need to exercise frequently and heavily to get many of its benefits. Physical conditioning—defined as an increase in maximal oxygen uptake—does require a certain duration and intensity of exercise, roughly twenty to thirty minutes, three times a week, at a level above 60 percent of your capacity. That may provide an extra degree of protection but don't give up on increased physical activity if you're unable or unwilling to do enough to attain conditioning.

For details beyond those given here, an excellent booklet published in 1974, "Exercise Your Way to Fitness and Heart Health" by Dr. L. R. Zohman, can be obtained from Best Foods (Englewood Cliffs, New Jersey 07632). For more about running and jogging, Dr. T. Kavanaugh's book, *The Healthy Heart Program* (Van Nostrand Reinhold, 1980), contains everything you'll ever need to know including how to get ready for a marathon. And of course, Dr. Kenneth Cooper's *The New Aerobics* (Bantam Books, 1976) has become a bible for many true believers in exercise.

The easiest and most available form of exercise is simply an increased level of walking, stair-climbing, package-carrying— all of the things you are now doing with the aid of cars, escalators, elevators, and golf carts. Park six blocks from your office and walk the distance, or better yet, ride a bicycle to work. Always walk up two flights of stairs and down four. Use a hand lawn mower.

With more leisure time, most Americans have been sitting longer and eating more. Watching professional sports and soap operas are our national pastimes and young people have given up sandlot baseball for Space Invaders. You should make a concerted effort to engage year-round in pleasurable, active sports—and if it's tennis, play singles.

If you are adequately motivated, start a regular program of isotonic exercise designed to bring you to physical fitness or conditioning (see Table 19, "Recommended Exercise Prescription"). The prescription involves the knowledge of the maximal heart rate that you can attain by physical exercise. This can be determined during a stress test or you can simply use the average values for your age (Figure 20). When you start your exercise program, use enough intensity to reach the 70 percent level, the bottom of the target zone. Once you are into your program, aim to keep the pulse in the target zone for twenty to thirty minutes, after a five-minute period of warm-up and followed by a five-minute cool-down.

Table 19: Recommended Exercise Prescription for Sedentary Adults

Type of Exercise: Walking, jogging, cycling, swimming

Intensity: Start at 60% to 70% of maximal heart rate
Achieve target zone between 70% and 85% of maximal heart rate

Duration: Start with 10- to 15-minute sessions
Progress to 20 to 60 minute sessions requiring at least 300 Kcal

Frequency: Start with sessions every other day
Remain at 3 days per week or progress to 5 days per week
Total weekly caloric expenditure at least 1000 Kcal.

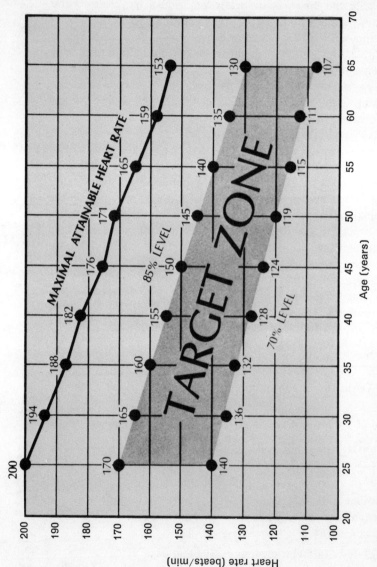

Figure 20. The maximal attainable heart rate during exercise decreases with age. The target zone is the 70% to 85% level that is the heart rate which should be reached and maintained for 20 minutes to achieve physical conditioning. (Source: Zohman, L. R., M.D., *Beyond Diet . . . Exercise Your Way to Fitness and Heart Health*, CPC International, Englewood Cliffs, N.J., 1974, p. 15)

The pulse should be taken, either at the wrist or in the neck, during and immediately upon stopping exercise. A 10-second count is enough, multiplied by six to obtain the minute pulse rate. As a rough guide to an adequate workout, you should still be able to talk but you should be breathless and sweating during the exercise. As you continue your exercise program, it will take more and more to keep you at the desired level. Once you've reached fitness, you will lose it rapidly if you cut your sessions below once a week. If you lay off, reduce the intensity and return gradually to your former level.

Regular isotonic exercise should make you look better and feel better, and it may also help you live longer. As always, though, the key is to do yourself no harm—so keep up the exercise as long as it makes you feel good; if for any reason you do not feel good while exercising, cut back on it until you find out why.

NINE

Stress and Personality Type

We now turn from the risk factors for cardiovascular disease that are, in general, easily measured—solid and firm—to one which may be as important as any of the rest but which is difficult to quantitate and to visualize: the way we handle stress. Not only is the stress factor hard to measure, but it may be impossible to change, so some tend to downplay its importance.

To begin with, there's no one definition of stress that is accepted by everyone. Most definitions involve the need to cope or adjust. One that is probably as good as any is that given by Dr. Herbert Benson in his book *The Relaxation Response*. He defines stress as "environmental conditions that require behavioral adjustment."[1]

We will consider two major aspects of the relationship between stress and heart disease: first, the effect of varying levels of external stress, such as in our jobs, marriages, socioeconomic status, and racial class; second, the effect of the different ways we react internally to whatever stress we face. The two obviously work together: a little external stress to a person who is easily provoked and full of hostility may cause more trouble than major stress to a person who is slow to anger and in full control of his emotions.

THE ROLE OF EXTERNAL STRESS

We are born with the ability to mobilize body defenses in response to whatever is perceived as a threat or stress. This "fight-or-flight" reaction prepares us to respond quickly and appropriately. But repeated exposure to too much stress or responses that are inappropriate and excessive may damage the heart and vasculature, leading to hypertension, atherosclerosis, and cardiovascular disease.

When an acute stress is perceived, a number of physiological responses are activated, mainly through an increased secretion of the hormone adrenaline:

- The heart beats faster and harder, causing the pulse and blood pressure to rise and increasing blood flow to vital organs.
- Breathing is deeper and faster.
- Intestinal activity slows (who needs gas at a time like this?).
- The body metabolism increases the supply of sugar and fatty acids to provide fuel for muscular activity.

The first and last of these responses—those by the heart and the metabolic machinery—can easily be seen to relate to the potential development of cardiovascular disease. Repeated bursts of increased heart action and constriction of blood vessels could set off a process leading to permanent hypertension. The combination of increased pressure against the vessel walls and higher levels of fatty acids could instigate the process of atherosclerosis.

Some believe that such repeated responses to acute stress or the persistent effects of chronic stress may be responsible for a great amount of disease. In particular, Canadian endocrinologist Dr. Hans Selye has long argued that most of human disease arises from "adaptation" to stress. Few go as far as Dr. Selye but most are willing to ascribe some of our troubles to misdirected responses to stress.

141

Table 20: The Rating of Stress in Adjusting to Change*

Event	Scale of Adjustment
Death of spouse	100
Divorce	73
Jail term	63
Death of close family member	63
Personal injury or illness	53
Marriage	50
Fired at work	47
Retirement	45
Pregnancy	40
Sex difficulties	39
Change to different line of work	36
Foreclosure of mortgage or loan	30
Son or daughter leaving home	29
Trouble with boss	23
Change in schools	20
Vacation	13
Christmas	12
Minor violations of the law	11

* From T. H. Holmes and R. H. J. Rahe, *Psychosomatic Research* 11 (1967): 216.

A number of relationships between stressful life events and cardiovascular disease have been described. One of the most famous is that of Drs. Thomas Holmes and Richard Rahl, who asked 394 people to give a numerical rating to the stress of adjusting to change, with marriage arbitrarily given 50 units (see Table 20). They then looked at the rates of sickness over a two-year period among more than five thousand people in comparison to the scores of the life changes they had experienced. The rates of developing an illness in two years were:

- 30 percent of those with low life change scores
- 50 percent of those with moderate scores
- 80 percent of those with high scores

Thus, stressful life changes are related to a greater likelihood of developing an illness. On the other hand, those who have strong social support seem to be protected. Married people have lower mortality rates than those who are single, widowed, or divorced. In keeping with the highest score in Table 20, given to death of spouse, rates of death and disease are particularly high during the first year of widowhood.

Perhaps the most striking demonstration of the values of social support in dealing with life's stresses comes from a nine-year follow-up of almost seven thousand people living in Alameda County, California, by Drs. Lisa Berkman and S. Leonard Syme. They found that people who lacked friends and family were almost three times more likely to die in those nine years than those with more extensive social and community contacts. This association was not related to socioeconomic status or various health practices such as smoking, drinking, or physical activity.

On the other hand, people in the lower socioeconomic classes and people who have less formal education are more likely to develop and die from coronary heart disease. This has been shown among men in various cities, including Sacramento, Oslo, and London. The latter group were divided into four grades of work status, from the highest (administrative) to the lowest ("other," men who were mainly unskilled manual workers). As reported by Drs. Geoffrey Rose and M. G. Marmot, the lowest socioeconomic class had almost four times the death rate from coronary heart disease over a seven-year period than did the highest (Figure 21). These different rates of death from heart disease were partly explained by known risk factors: the men in the lower classes smoked more, exercised less, were more overweight, and had higher blood pressures. But after taking all of these factors into account, most of the differences remained unexplained. Presumably the dis-

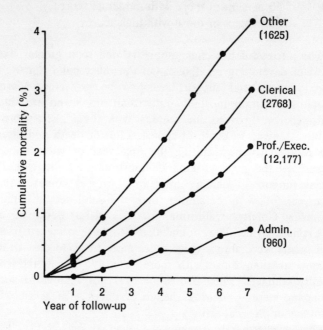

Figure 21. The cumulative mortality from coronary heart disease over 7 years among 17,530 London civil servants aged 40 to 64, classified by their employment grade. (Source: Rose, G., and Marmot, M. G., *British Heart Journal* 45 [1981]: 13)

crepancy was not related to differences in health care since all of these men were civil servants who had free and equal access to medical services.

The assumption from all of these studies is that those who are poor and uneducated are more subject to stress than those who are affluent and educated, that the former are therefore more likely to develop cardiovascular disease. Drs. Rose and Marmot found that the death rate for heart disease has been steadily rising for the lower social classes in England since 1931 but that it has been stable since 1951 for those in the upper classes. Remember, too, that hypertension is more

144

prevalent among blacks and other social groups under high levels of stress.

Not all researchers acknowledge this inverse relation between socioeconomic status and heart disease. After all, people who approach the top of the ladder of success are usually thought to be exposed to *more* stress, not less. Obviously, the climb may be stressful but those who get to the top do seem to be protected, not just from heart disease but from all causes of mortality. If being listed in *Who's Who* can be accepted as a reasonably good measure of success, most of those who are listed, with the exception of journalists, have lower death rates than the general population (Table 21). Even politicians, who should be among the most highly stressed people in our society, had lower death rates. Presidents of the United States, senators, and congressmen have a much longer life-expectancy than the rest of us.

Perhaps the figures would be different for those who weren't successful enough to be listed in *Who's Who*. But remember the "good news" described earlier in chapter 1: death rates

Table 21: Comparative Mortality of Prominent Men Listed in Who's Who*

Vocational Group	Mortality Rate Relative to General Population (100%)
All groups	70%
Scientists	55%
College professors	61%
Clergymen	62%
Business executives	71%
Physicians	78%
Government officials	81%
Journalists	134%

* From *Statistical Bulletin* (January–March 1979): 8.

from heart disease have been decreasing in the United States since 1968, despite Vietnam, Watergate, inflation, urban decay, and all the other aspects of increasing stress in all of our lives. This takes us to the next aspect of stress: how we respond may be even more important than the level of stress to which we are exposed.

THE EFFECT OF INTERNAL REACTIONS TO STRESS: TYPE A BEHAVIOR

In 1896, the famous physician Sir William Osler noted that the young coronary-heart-disease (angina) patient was typically "the robust, the vigorous in mind and body, the keen and ambitious man, the indicator of whose engine is always set 'full speed ahead'."[2]

Osler was probably describing a person with the Type A behavior pattern, characterized in the late 1950s by Drs. Meyer Friedman and Ray Rosenman as having these traits:

- Intense striving for achievement
- Competitiveness
- Being easily provoked
- Impatience
- Time urgency; preoccupation with deadlines
- Abruptness of gestures and speech
- Overcommitment to vocation or profession
- Excesses of drive and hostility[3]

Those who are Type B have an opposite pattern of behavior—relaxed, unhurried, less easily provoked, smoothly modulated speech and gesture patterns. This distinction was first made during a personal interview but now it's most often based upon a questionnaire, usually the Jenkins Activity Survey (JAS), which can be graded by computer.

Actually, you can tell with a high degree of accuracy if you are Type A or B just by self-assessment. The self-ratings using the checklist of adjectives shown in Table 22 were closely

146

Table 22: Checklist of Adjectives for Type A Self-Assessment*

Percent of Accuracy	Characteristic	Uncharacteristic
100	Aggressive, hurried	Easy-going
90–100	Active, alert, ambitious, assertive, dominant, energetic, hostile, impatient, irritable, quick	Calm, relaxed
80–90	Determined, forceful, impulsive, restless	Mild, slow, patient, unambitious
70–80	Argumentative, bossy, excitable, industrious, persistent, tense	Leisurely, quiet, reflective, unexcitable

* Reprinted by permission of the publisher from "Self-ratings of Type A (Coronary Prone) Adults: Do Type A's Know They Are Type A's," by S. Herman, J. A. Blumenthal, G. M. Black, and M. A. Chesney, in *Psychosomatic Medicine* 43 (1981): 407. Copyright 1981 by The American Gastroenterological Association.

related to the classification obtained by a traditional structured interview.

The number of Type A persons in different groups ranges anywhere from 15 percent to 80 percent. About half of urban, middle-class, middle-aged American men are Type A. There are more Type A's in occupations with higher prestige and among people with higher levels of education. Most of the studies on Type A and B have been done on middle-class American men, so we're less sure of the prevalence among women, blacks, and other groups.

A large number of studies have confirmed Rosenman and Friedman's findings that Type A men have at least twice the

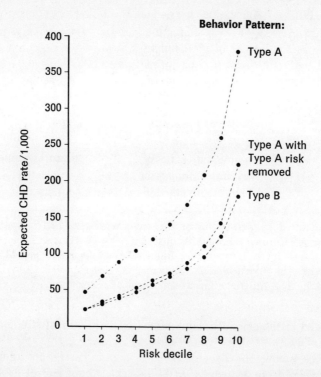

Figure 22. The expected death rate from coronary heart disease in 8.5 years for 50- to 59-year-old men classified by their behavior pattern and ranked by their risk decile (their degree of other cardiovascular risks, including age, cholesterol, blood pressure, and smoking status). The higher the risk decile, the higher the degree of risk. (Source: Brand, R. J. *et al.*, "Multivariance Prediction of Coronary Heart Disease in the Western Collaborative Group Study Compared to the Findings of the Framingham Study," *Circulation* 53 [1976]: 348. By permission of the American Heart Association, Inc.)

likelihood of developing coronary heart disease. Their primary research was done with more than three thousand men employed in ten companies in California who were studied for eight and a half years (Figure 22). This group of 50- to 59-year-old men included some whose initial Type A pattern was "removed" by a program of behavior modification. Note that their rate of heart disease fell to almost equal that of the Type B men. Based on this study, the authors predicted that as many as 31 percent of the deaths from heart disease could be attributed to the Type A behavior pattern.

Confirmation and expansion of these findings have come from the Framingham study, reported by Suzanne Haynes and coworkers. They found that women, too, who were Type A had twice the rate of coronary heart disease whether they were housewives or otherwise employed.[4] Furthermore, they found that the association between Type A behavior and coronary disease among men was present in those with white-collar jobs but not in those with blue-collar jobs. The risk for heart disease was also increased among those with suppressed hostility (not showing or discussing anger), work overload, and frequent job promotions. Once again, the Type A pattern was an independent risk when all other known risk factors were accounted for.

Type A people do not necessarily have a greater feeling of anxiety or depression. Being Type A is not the same as enduring "stress," nor is it an unpleasant feeling. Nonetheless, the Type A pattern, like chronic painful emotions, probably works through the nervous system to invoke greater hormonal and metabolic responses to various stresses. When stressed, Type A people have been shown to release more adrenaline and to have a greater rise in blood pressure. A great deal more work needs to be done to uncover the manner by which Type A behavior is translated into cardiovascular risk.

CHANGING TYPE A TO TYPE B

Friedman and Rosenman offer these suggestions as "drills" to change Type A behavior:

- Reinforce non-Type A behavior: instead of business lunches, take lunchtime walks in the park, browse through bookstores, and so on.
- Avoid situations that elicit feelings of time pressure and hostility: do not wear a watch, don't make a list of "things to do today," don't schedule back-to-back activities.
- Use self-control techniques such as biofeedback, the relaxation response, TM, or yoga.[5]

Another proponent of behavioral change, Dr. Robert Eliot, has suggested that we should act as though we have six months to live: ridding ourselves of all unnecessary and unproductive activities, delegating work, saying no, establishing priorities. Thereby, he suggests, it is possible to "convert a thin-skinned, extremely sensitive, over-reactive person into a thick-skinned, more resilient, less reactive human being."[6]

Maybe so, but scientific proof of such conversions is almost totally lacking, as is any real evidence that if one becomes a "non-Type A," cardiovascular risk will diminish. If the Type A person is also hypertensive, a program of relaxation training may at least lower the blood pressure even if it doesn't reduce the Type A behavior pattern.[7]

One of the problems inherent in attempts to change Type A people is that in our society Type A behavior is usually rewarded with job promotion, increased income, and other indices of success. Thus, most Type A people don't want to change and they deny their Type A behaviors.

At the least, those who are Type A should receive all the protection that is available by reduction of the other, less socially desirable, risk factors. No one enjoys high blood pressure or high blood cholesterol levels and cigarette smoking is becoming socially unacceptable.

CHAPTER

TEN

Alcohol

Now that you've been asked to cut down on calories, saturated fat, and salt, take pills for hypertension, increase your level of physical activity, and not wear a watch (can that really help correct your Type A behavior?), we've come to one strategy to reduce your cardiovascular risk that you'll probably enjoy: drink a moderate amount of alcohol regularly. There is now very convincing evidence that the regular consumption of about an ounce of alcohol a day will reduce your chances for developing heart disease. However, let me clearly and unequivocally say that heavy alcohol consumption—more than three or four ounces a day—will hurt you, physically, mentally, and socially. Heavy alcohol intake will kill you well before your appointed time. My point is that, in *moderation,* the use of alcohol will probably reduce your cardiovascular risk.

Some strongly oppose this view and believe that drinking should not be encouraged in any way, in any amount, for any reason. Some of this opposition is based on religious grounds, some on the feeling that it may add to the terrible personal and social burdens already caused by those who abuse alcohol. To those who feel this way, let me offer these rebuttals:

· I sincerely doubt that anyone who is encouraged to drink one or, at the most, two ounces of alcohol a day will be converted into an alcoholic—unless there is some predisposition toward the disease. Almost 90 percent of all U.S. adults have drunk alcohol. Unlike cigarettes, which are so highly addicting, the exposure to alcohol rarely leads to abuse. I am reminded of the evidence that alcoholism was always rare among Jews until recent years when they have discarded many of their traditional practices. One of the reasons given for this rare abuse of alcohol was their exposure to small amounts at family religious ceremonies, where drinking a few glasses of wine and an occasional schnapps was encouraged. Alcohol was a familiar part of their lives and did not tend to assume undue importance for them.

· We do not know why perhaps 10 percent of those who drink start their progressive fall into alcoholism. Complex psychological, social, and perhaps physical differences presumably mark them as susceptible. Encouragement of unlimited and widespread consumption of alcohol might cause more to become alcoholics. Obviously, this is not intended—and the distinction can be made.

· My recommendation of moderate alcohol consumption can be compared to my attitude toward physical activity. I believe that some physical exercise is good for everyone, but it only need be taken in moderation. Only a few who take that advice will go on into progressively heavier exercise. Those who go beyond, into 26-, 50-, and 100-mile marathons, should in no way be likened to alcoholics—but maybe they too have become addicted.

· Most important, we have strong evidence that *regular, moderate* alcohol use will improve our health status. Both teetotalers and heavy drinkers have more cardiovascular mortality than those who drink moderately.

Dr. Raymond Pearl, the same physician who first identified the danger of cigarette smoking in 1934, was the first to recognize, in 1926, that moderate drinkers have a lower mortality rate than either abstainers or heavy drinkers. In the last few years, an impressive body of epidemiological evidence has come forth, consistently demonstrating lower cardiovascular risks in those who drink one to two ounces of alcohol daily. This evidence has come from such diverse groups as enrollees in the Kaiser-Permanente health plan in Oakland-San Francisco, in Japanese men living in Hawaii, and in British civil servants in London (Table 23).

The data from this latter study, reported by Dr. Marmot and associates, are particularly straightforward and fairly representative of the rest of the evidence. They show about a

---

Table 23: Studies That Have Shown Less Risk for Coronary Heart Disease with Moderate Alcohol Intake

Kaiser-Permanente enrollees	(Klatsky, 1974, 1981)
Framingham, Mass., population	(Stason, 1976)
Japanese men in Hawaii	(Yano, 1977)
Boston men	(Hennekens, 1978)
Yugoslavian men	(Kozarevic, 1980)
British civil servants	(Marmot, 1981)
Employed men in Chicago	(Dyer, 1981)
Young women in Boston	(Rosenberg, 1981)

153

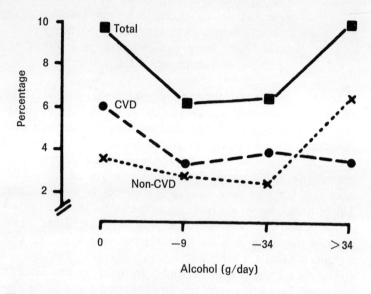

Figure 23. The percentage rates of death from all causes (total), cardiovascular diseases (CVD), and noncardiovascular (non-CVD) causes according to daily average alcohol consumption in 10 years among 1,422 civil servants in London. (Source: Marmot, M. G. *et al., Lancet* 1 [1981]: 578)

one-third lower death rate for cardiovascular disease and total mortality among those who drink an average of from 9 to 34 grams of alcohol a day (Figure 23). This corresponds to from 10 to 40 milliliters of pure alcohol. Most of the studies listed in Table 23 show a similar reduction in risk for coronary heart disease, in the range of one-third to one-half less, among those who drink an average of one-half to two ounces of alcohol per day. So it takes relatively little alcohol, the amount present in one to two beers, glasses of wine, or mixed drinks per day, to derive the potential benefit.

The total mortality goes back up in those who drink more

154

than an average of 34 grams of alcohol a day (Figure 23). Others find mortality to increase only with a somewhat higher intake, but all agree that those who drink heavily die earlier. Their increased mortality does not include more atherosclerotic coronary heart disease, but does involve liver disease, heart failure, cancer, automobile accidents, and other trauma.

In addition to these individual studies, nationwide rates of death from atherosclerotic heart disease (ASHD) are also closely related to per capita alcohol consumption.[2] Finns and Americans, high in death rates from ASHD, are relatively low in alcohol consumption. On the other hand, the wine-loving, heavier-drinking French and Italians have much less coronary mortality. However, they do not have a longer life-expectancy than we do, presumably because other diseases associated with such high alcohol use are more prevalent. The Japanese, despite a very low average alcohol intake, have the world's lowest death rate from coronary heart disease. Presumably their very low saturated-fat intake and blood cholesterol protect them, as noted in Chapter 5.

Why do those who drink some alcohol have less atherosclerotic heart disease, specifically myocardial infarctions? The exact reasons are not known but three factors are probably responsible:

1. Alcohol increases the amount of the protective form of blood cholesterol, the HDL cholesterol (Figure 24). As shown in these data, increasing alcohol intake progressively raises HDL while lowering the LDL form.

2. Moderate amounts of alcohol may lower the blood pressure. The evidence is not as conclusive or uniform as with HDL cholesterol but some population studies show a similar U-shaped curve for blood pressure and alcohol: higher blood pressures in those who abstain or drink heavily, lower in those who drink one to two ounces per day.

155

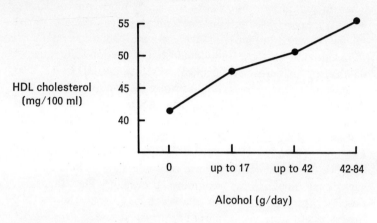

Figure 24. One of the effects of increasing consumption of alcohol, in grams per day, is shown to be an increase in the HDL-cholesterol, which is thought to protect against heart disease. These data are from a study involving 4,000 men and women in 10 different places in the United States and Canada. (Source: Gordon, T. *et al., Circulation* 64, supp. 3 [1981]: 63)

3. Psychological stress may be lessened by moderate alcohol use. There is no good information about this but it seems logical.

In most of these studies, the protection associated with moderate amounts of alcohol was independent of other known risk factors. It is true that, in some groups, abstainers were sometimes heavier smokers or more obese, but the alcohol effect is not dependent on having less of the other risk factors.

However it happens, *regular* consumption of *moderate* amounts of alcohol seems to offer protection. Notice again: regular and moderate. The evidence that it needs to be regular

---

Table 24: The Alcohol Content of Various Drinks

One drink　　= one-half ounce or 15 milliliters of alcohol

Distilled spirits (whiskey, vodka, rum, gin)

　80 proof　　= 40% alcohol
　1½ ounces　= 18 milliliters of alcohol

Wine　　　　= 12% alcohol
　4 ounces　　= 14.4 milliliters of alcohol

Beer　　　　 = 4.5% alcohol
　12 ounces　= 16.2 milliliters of alcohol

Therefore, to consume 30 milliliters (one ounce) of alcohol per day, you'll need to drink:

　　2 mixed drinks containing 1½-ounce jigger
　　2　4-ounce glasses of wine or
　　2　12-ounce bottles of beer

---

is not especially strong, but we've seen considerable evidence for the moderate amount.

In one study from Milwaukee, X-rays were used to determine the degrees of narrowing of the coronary blood vessels in a group of men with heart disease.[3] The degree of narrowing was then related to both the amount and pattern of the patients' drinking behavior. Those who drank in binges, two or more times their average consumption at one sitting, had more extensive narrowing of their coronary blood vessels. We need much more such evidence concerning the pattern of alcohol intake and the reduction of cardiovascular risk. But it certainly makes good sense to drink only a little at a time. In large amounts, alcohol can only be considered a poison, destroying brain and liver cells, damaging the heart muscle, and impairing all body functions, including sexual performance; and of course there are the many dangers resulting from drunkenness.

As to the quantity of alcohol needed for reduction of cardio-vascular risk, it takes only a small amount, well below the quantity that impairs brain or other body functions. If the amounts shown in Table 24 ("The Alcohol Content of Various Drinks") are consumed with food over an hour or two, no obvious or hidden ill effects should be experienced. Which form of drink you prefer is irrelevant as far as the reduction of risk is concerned: it's the alcohol that does the trick. You may need to consider calories, since you'll get more of them with beer and the mixers often used for cocktails (see Table 14, page 110).

I would like to add, as a final word, that most medical experts, even though they accept the evidence of lower risk with moderate alcohol consumption, do not go along with these recommendations. The director of the Framingham study, Dr. William Castelli, concluded in 1979 that "with 17 million alcoholics in this country," the prescription of alcohol as a prophylactic against coronary disease "is a message for which this country is not yet ready."[4] His is the prevailing opinion, but I believe that mine does not go against the one rule we must all follow in advocating widespread preventive measures: do no harm.

ELEVEN

Sex and Hormones

Women in the United States live, on an average, eight years longer than men, reflecting less atherosclerosis and only about half as much mortality from cardiovascular disease.[1] As the patterns of women's lives have altered, both beneficial and deleterious effects have been seen—among the latter some factors that threaten to reduce or abolish their relative protection from premature heart disease. But up to the present, the fact of being male has been the best documented and the least understood risk factor for incurring cardiovascular disease.

Are there any logical explanations for the much lower rate of heart disease in women? Yes and no. Their relative invulnerability before menopause can be explained by their lower exposure to a number of the known risk factors. They have less hypertension; they have a more favorable blood-lipid profile with lower levels of LDL cholesterol and higher levels of HDL cholesterol; and, although they are rapidly destroying this advantage, they smoke less.

But after age 50, during their postmenopausal years, women tend to lose their favorable risk-profile and develop more hypertension and higher cholesterols than men. They also begin incurring more heart disease, though their relative risk remains well below that of men. Among the 2,873 women in the

159

Framingham population who were studied for twenty-four years, no premenopausal women had a heart attack; but among those aged 50 to 54, twenty-five episodes of coronary disease were noted.

Among the Framingham group, an ominous indication of increasing danger for women was also noted: those who took jobs outside the home had a higher rate of heart disease (7.8 percent) compared to housewives (5.4 percent). Moreover, women performing clerical jobs had almost twice the rate of heart disease (10.6 percent). We're not sure of the reasons for this, and this higher rate has not been noted among all groups of women working outside the home. But without question, as more women adopt bad habits—in particular cigarette smoking—they will be taking on more risk for heart disease.

One explanation for the higher rates of heart disease among women after menopause is that premenopausal women have greater levels of the female hormone, estrogen, and this level falls after menopause. In light of this observation, large numbers of men were given estrogens in the 1950s and 1960s in hopes of reducing their high rate of heart disease. It didn't work; in fact, these men developed even more heart disease, along with a loss of their sexual drive. This was not so surprising in view of what we now know about the multiple effects of estrogens, which sometimes include:

- A rise in blood pressure.
- An increased tendency for the blood to clot.
- An increased tightness (spasm) with the coronary arteries.

These effects will be considered further when we discuss the use of oral contraceptives. Along with the potentially harmful effects, estrogens cause at least one beneficial effect: they raise the level of HDL cholesterol.

The relations between female hormones and heart disease are complicated and poorly understood. There is an obvious paradox: young women with high levels of natural estrogen have

160

little heart disease; older men exposed to estrogens develop more heart disease. A possible explanation is a difference in the effects of estrogens at different times of life—in the young, the higher levels of HDL cholesterol induced by the estrogen would decrease the development of the fatty plaques that lead to atherosclerosis; but when estrogens are given to older men, who already have some atherosclerosis causing roughening of the artery walls, the greater tendency for the blood to clot would favor the development of obstructions (thromboses) at the rough places which lead to heart attacks.

Beyond these multiple effects of female hormones, there may be a very simple explanation for the lesser vulnerability of young women. Young women lose about three to four ounces of blood every month by menstruation. As a result, they have, normally, about 20 percent fewer red cells and 20 percent less total volume of blood—even compared to men of the same size. Perhaps this lesser amount of blood exerts less pressure against their blood vessels and less strain upon their hearts. It sounds too simple, but data show an immediate threefold increase in the rates of coronary heart disease in young women who have a hysterectomy and thereby quit menstruating but who still have ovaries and normal amounts of female hormones. Thus, though they are premenopausal as far as hormone production is concerned, their cessation of menses seems to bring on cardiovascular disease.[2]

THE RISK OF ADDED ESTROGENS

Another reason that a functioning uterus may protect against cardiovascular disease has been suggested: the uterus produces a hormone, prostacyclin, which keeps blood platelets from sticking together, thereby reducing the tendency for blood to clot.[3] More about prostacyclin will be covered in the next chapter.

Although we may never unravel the male-female differences in vulnerability to cardiovascular disease, we do know that today millions of women are taking extra amounts of female hormones and thereby may be exposing themselves to potential hazards. These hormones are being taken by younger women for contraception and by older women for prevention of the effects of aging.

Almost all contraceptive pills currently used contain a combination of estrogen and a derivative of the other major female hormone, progesterone. The estrogen is the major contraceptive, the progesterone derivative acting primarily to modulate the menstrual bleeding that follows the monthly withdrawal of the estrogen.

Women who take a contraceptive pill have a higher risk for heart disease, stroke, and blood clots in the legs. The increase in their *relative risk,* compared to women of the same age who do not take the pill, is definite and considerable (see Table 25). This higher risk probably reflects the various cardiovascular alterations described previously. Notice that even women who ceased using oral contraceptives continued to have a higher relative risk, suggesting that some of the estrogen-induced damages are irreversible.

As impressive as these statistics are, they should not be taken as proof that use of the pill will cause harm to a large number of women. These additional points should be considered:

1. The pill is the most effective contraceptive now available. Prevention of unwanted pregnancies

---

Table 25: Relative Risk of Mortality by Oral Contraceptive Use*

Cause of Death	Relative Risk	
	CURRENT USERS	FORMER USERS
All heart diseases	7.3	4.6
Coronary artery disease	6.4	2.0
Cerebrovascular diseases	2.0	3.6
All circulatory diseases	4.0	4.3

* From Royal College of General Practitioners, "Oral Contraceptive Study," *Lancet* 1 (1981): 541.

thereby saves the lives of some women who would die from spontaneously occurring diseases of pregnancy or from complications of abortion.

2. The *absolute risk* is still quite minor. The number of heart attacks and strokes occurring in nonpill users in their 20's and 30's is very small. Therefore, even though pill users have a four- to sevenfold increase in their relative risk, the total number of serious complications remains small.

3. Most of the risk from the pill occurs in those who are over age 35 and who also smoke cigarettes (Table 26). A pill-taking woman under age 35 who does not smoke has only a 1 in 77,000 chance for trouble; a pill-taking woman over age 45 who smokes has a 1 in 500 chance.

Overall, the estrogen-containing oral contraceptive pill remains the most effective and safest form of temporary birth control for a large number of young women who need or wish to prevent pregnancy. Some may prefer other devices (IUD, condom, diaphragm) which have higher rates of failure. Those who no longer want temporary birth control but permanent pregnancy prevention should use sterilization. (And, by the

---

Table 26: The Estimated Excess Risk of Pill Use*
(excess annual death rates)

	NONSMOKERS	SMOKERS
Under age 35	1:77,000	1:10,000
Age 35–44	1:6,700	1:2,000
Over age 45	1:2,500	1:500

---

* From Royal College of General Practitioners, "Oral Contraceptive Study," *Lancet* 1 (1981): 541.

way, a report that vasectomized men have a higher subsequent rate of heart disease has not been verified.)

Women are also using estrogens after menopause in hopes of preventing or delaying some of the effects of the aging process and certain beneficial effects of postmenopausal estrogens have been shown. These include prevention of:

· Menopausal hot flashes.
· Dryness and irritation of the vaginal skin.
· Thinning of the bones.

The last of these, known as osteoporosis, is a serious problem in at least 25 percent of women as they grow older, leading to collapsed vertebrae and broken hips following even minimal trauma. More and more evidence has shown that estrogen use, along with adequate calcium intake and continued physical activity, will prevent much of this bone thinning.

However, women taking estrogens after menopause who have not had a hysterectomy thereby expose themselves to a greater likelihood of cancer of the endometrium, the lining of the uterus. Fortunately, the use of a progesterone derivative with the estrogen appears to reduce that risk, though it may cause menstrual bleeding to persist.

It is also encouraging that data show the use of postmenopausal estrogen does not appear to increase the risk for cardiovascular disease and may actually decrease the risk. In at least four studies involving large numbers of women, the relative risk for death from a heart attack has been found to be reduced as much as 60 percent among those who are taking estrogens.[4]

Why the protection? We really do not know. But recall the differences in the effects of increasing the amount of estrogens in younger women and in older women. The younger start with considerably higher levels of HDL cholesterol, the older with much lower levels. Moreover, the amount and potency of the estrogen given for postmenopausal therapy is usually less than that needed for contraception. In addition, a reverse effect upon blood cholesterol occurs in the older users of estrogen (Figure 25). The younger oral-contraceptive users

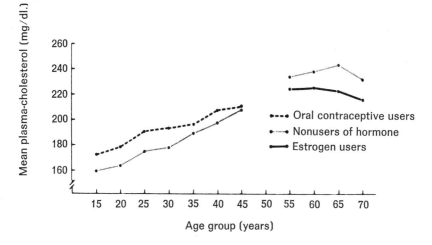

Figure 25. The average plasma cholesterol levels in younger women who used estrogen-containing oral contraceptives (---) or postmenopausal women taking estrogens (———), compared to nonusers of the hormone at similar ages (. . . . .). (Source: Wallace, R. B. *et al., Lancet* 2 [1979]: 111)

had a rise in total cholesterol, the older, postmenopausal users, a fall. Whatever the reason, it seems safe, as regards cardiovascular health, for older women to take estrogens.

Finally, a brief word about erotic pleasures. Sexual intercourse between two consenting partners is safe as long as neither harbors a venereal disease. It is true that one's blood pressure and pulse rise along with one's passion and, during orgasm, both may be quite high. But the effect is transient, and it's no more of a strain than a mile jog. One last point—if you're concerned, as during convalescence after a heart attack—the rises in both blood pressure and pulse during orgasm were found to be similar whoever was on top. If caution is advised, try lovemaking without orgasm first and then a slow, relaxed session of intercourse with both partners lying on their sides.

TWELVE

Where Do We Go from Here?: Putting the Pieces Together

We've now covered the important risk factors for cardio-vascular disease. Practical advice has been provided to help you reduce your risks. But let's consider an overall perspective—you can't do everything at once and you may be confused as to how much you should attempt.

A Little Bit of Many Factors

It's unlikely that you have a high level of any one risk factor. Rather, if you're a typical American, you will have a slightly elevated cholesterol and blood pressure and you'll smoke about a pack of cigarettes a day. But your combination of risks, each in fairly small degrees, adds up to a considerable increase in overall risk (see Table 27, "Equivalent Risks for Coronary Heart Disease"). As shown on the last line in Table 27, if you are a 50-year-old man you run as high a risk for a heart attack in five or twenty years by having a slightly elevated cholesterol (250) and blood pressure (96 diastolic) and a daily habit of thirty cigarettes as that same man with a much higher degree of any one risk.

These various risks tend to multiply each other's effects (Figure 26). The Framingham data for a 45-year-old man show

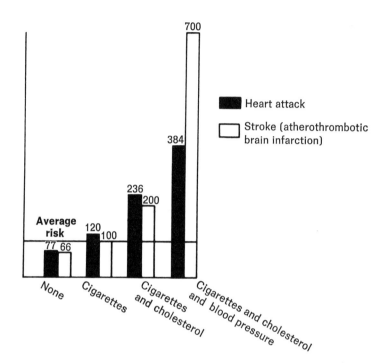

Figure 26. The risk for a heart attack or stroke in a 45-year-old male with none, one, two, or three major risk factors for cardiovascular disease, based upon the Framingham study. Cigarettes = one pack per day; cholesterol = 310 mg/dl; blood pressure = 180 mm Hg systolic. (Source: Framingham, Massachusetts, Heart Study)

the risk for a heart attack to be five times greater and more than ten times greater for a stroke when all three of the major risk factors are present.

The message should be clear—you must be concerned even about small degrees of each risk, particularly if you have more

167

Table 27: Equivalent Risks for Coronary Heart Disease in a 50-Year-Old Man

Serum Cholesterol (mg/ 100 ml.)		Smoking (Cigarettes/ day)		Diastolic Blood Pressure (mm/Hg)		Risks for Coronary Heart Disease in 5 Years	in 20 Years
400	+	0	+	80	=	9%	43%
225	+	60	+	80	=	9%	43%
225	+	0	+	125	=	9%	43%
250	+	30	+	96	=	9%	43%

than one. On the other hand, you can relax some if you have only a mild degree of one risk—but even then, why not be good to yourself and reduce your risk even further?

The Need to Choose Your Parents

Whatever your current status, you need to look at your family history. If parents, grandparents, aunts, uncles, or siblings suffered from cardiovascular disease, it's more likely that you will too. Sometimes the reason is obvious: hypertension, hyper-cholesterolemia, and diabetes are often hereditary, being passed on in the genes from one generation to the next. But often no specific hereditary connection can be identified. The propensity toward shared risks may reflect a common environment and cultural preferences. Whatever the reason, be even more careful if others in your family have or have had premature heart disease.

In the same light, if you are at risk, be sure your children are protected by proper diet, exercise, and medical surveillance.

Coffee, Tea, and Other Beverages

One additional aspect of your and your family's diet should be considered since Americans consume more caffeine than any other people in the world. The caffeine present in coffee, tea, and many soft drinks has been accused of causing considerable mischief. One report from Boston in 1973 claimed that those who drank one to five cups of coffee a day had a 60 percent increase in heart attacks. But since then, numerous, more carefully documented reports have shown no independent risk from even larger amounts of coffee. One problem with the first report was the failure to consider that heavy coffee drinkers tend to be heavy smokers as well.

Some people do respond adversely to the mild stimulatory effect of caffeine upon the central nervous system and heart. Other than keeping you awake if you drink it before retiring or causing an occasional fast heartbeat, it's unusual to see trouble even with heavy caffeine intake.

If you want to keep your caffeine intake down, consider how much is in six ounces of these beverages:

Decaffeinated coffee	3 milligrams
Cocoa	10 milligrams
Dr. Pepper	30 milligrams
Coca-Cola	31 milligrams
Leaf tea, 5 min. brew	41 milligrams
Brewed coffee, dripolator	180 milligrams

Less Than an Aspirin a Day May Keep the Doctor Away

And lastly, there is a reasonably good chance that we may reduce our risk for cardiovascular disease by taking a small amount of aspirin intermittently. The evidence is still fragmentary and based more upon what we know goes on in the body than upon large-scale, experimental proof of protection.

Your body makes a family of hormones called prostaglandins (the first was discovered in fluid from the prostate gland). These prostaglandins affect a large number of different body processes and either deficits or surpluses of one or more of them may be responsible for a variety of diseases. One prostaglandin hormone called prostacyclin is made within your blood vessel wall and it acts to keep the small blood vessels

169

dilated and to prevent the clumping of tiny cells in your blood (called platelets) which are responsible for the start of a blood clot. Another prostaglandin, called thromboxane, is made in these same platelets. It does just the reverse of prostacyclin, acting to constrict the small blood vessels and to encourage the platelets to clump together and start a blood clot.

These latter functions of thromboxane help platelets do what they are thought to be responsible for—the formation of blood clots to stop bleeding at exposed sites. By constricting the small blood vessels and starting the process of blood clotting, they would help stop the flow of blood from a cut or wound.

But these same effects could be harmful if they were activated within the blood vessels, as at the roughened site of an atherosclerotic plaque in an artery wall. Thereby a blood clot would start and lead to an obstruction of the blood flow (thrombosis). Such a process, within the blood vessels, may be responsible for heart attacks and strokes. Thus, just as we have both good and bad forms of cholesterol, we have both good (prostacyclin) and bad (thromboxane) forms of prostaglandins.

A few years ago, a remarkable effect of our most popular drug, aspirin, was discovered: it prevented the formation of these prostaglandins. And then an even more remarkable discovery was made: a very small amount of aspirin would block the formation of the bad prostaglandin (thromboxane) and not interfere with the formation of the good prostaglandin (prostacyclin). It only takes about one milligram of aspirin for each kilogram of body weight or about one-half milligram per pound every three to four days to accomplish this balancing act. That comes out to be about seventy-five milligrams of aspirin for an average adult man—just the amount found in one baby aspirin.

Larger amounts of aspirin, two to four adult-sized tablets a day (each with 300 milligrams of aspirin), have been shown to reduce the recurrence of heart attacks and strokes (the latter in men but not in women). The smaller amounts have not been shown to prevent any disease in anyone. But the intriguing effect of the smaller dose to remove the potentially harmful thromboxane while leaving the protective prostacyclin has prompted me to take one baby aspirin every Monday and Thursday morning for the last two years.

I do not know if this will prevent heart attacks and strokes. I do know that it will change some processes in the body which should help prevent these cardiovascular catastrophes. And I also know that, unless you are allergic to aspirin, that small dose will not do you any harm.

More Conservative Advice

Whether aspirin helps or not, you should do those things that have proved or are highly likely to be proved helpful in reducing the risk of cardiovascular disease. The Revised U.S. Dietary Goals of 1978 (see Table 28) are a good place to start. Add some regular isotonic exercise, a little alcohol, and a

---

Table 28: Revised United States Dietary Goals (1978)

To avoid overweight, consume only as much energy (calories) as is expended; if overweight, decrease energy intake, and increase energy expenditure.

Increase the consumption of complex carbohydrates and "naturally occurring" sugars from about 28% of energy intake to about 48% of energy intake.

Reduce the consumption of refined and processed sugars by about 45% to account for about 10% of total energy intake.

Reduce overall fat consumption from approximately 40% to about 30% of energy intake.

Reduce saturated fat consumption to account for about 10% of total energy intake; and balance that with polyunsaturated and monounsaturated fats, which should account for about 10% of energy intake each.

Reduce cholesterol consumption to about 300 mg per day.

Limit the intake of sodium by reducing the intake of salt to about 5 grams per day.

171

touch of aspirin, and you should live a longer life, free of the major diseases that now cause most of our disability and premature death.

Which of these strategies you want to start with depends upon your overall risk status, your psychological makeup, and your current life situation. You may, having decided to straighten out your messed-up health status, go after all the risks you carry. If you've got the willpower, go to it. Some find the full press is more effective and in the long run easier than picking off one piece at a time. Here are a couple of suggested strategies:

- You are a heavy smoker, 30 pounds overweight, and moderately hypertensive (blood pressure = 160/105): Start with a lower-calorie, lower-sodium diet and an exercise program. But leave the cigarettes alone; if you lose 20 pounds, your blood pressure will likely come down and you'll then be in much better shape to fight the cigarettes, particularly the tendency to gain weight when you quit.
- You have a high cholesterol, 25 pounds of extra weight, an elevated blood pressure, and an average alcohol consumption of a 6-pack of beer a day: Start with a lower-calorie, lower-saturated fat, lower-sodium diet and cut the beer to 2 or 3 per day. The diet may straighten out the blood pressure, cholesterol, and weight. The beer needn't be stopped, but 3 fewer a day will protect your liver and other vital organs and cut your calories by almost 500 calories a day.

Obviously your situation may involve one of a hundred different combinations. As a general guideline, starting a lower-calorie, lower-saturated fat, lower-sodium diet with increased physical activity is a good approach for almost everyone. Working on smoking, Type A personality, drug treatment of mild hypertension, and alcohol may then be more effective and easier to accomplish.

One strategy you may prefer is to start with a serious isotonic exercise program: most regular joggers lose weight, cut down cigarettes, and probably lower their blood pressure and raise their HDL cholesterol levels. If your Type A personality pattern changes along with all the rest, you may agree that jogging is the quickest way to improved cardiovascular health.

Whatever you do, be sensible. Use a game plan that has a reasonable chance of working and don't give up if you fall behind repeatedly. Success rarely comes from the first try and you shouldn't look upon yourself as a failure if you don't accomplish all you're after. In the meantime, remember to take that baby aspirin every Monday and Thursday.

When all is said and done, it's your life and you're the only one who can make the difference. Here's to your health.

Notes

CHAPTER 2

1. Geoffrey Rose, "Strategy of Prevention: Lessons from Cardio-vascular Disease," *British Medical Journal* 282 (1981): 1847.

CHAPTER 5

1. I. Hjermann *et al.,* "Effect of Diet and Smoking Intervention on the Incidence of Coronary Heart Disease," *Lancet* 2 (1981): 1303.

2. Ancel Keys, *Seven Countries: A Multivariate Analysis of Death and Coronary Heart Disease* (Cambridge, Mass.: Harvard University Press, 1980), p. 122.

CHAPTER 6

1. Ancel Keys, "Overweight, Obesity, Coronary Heart Disease and Mortality," *Nutrition Reviews* 38 (1980): 297.

2. Faith T. Fitzgerald, "The Problem of Obesity." Reproduced with permission from the *Annual Review of Medicine,* Volume 32, p. 221, © 1981 by Annual Reviews Inc.

3. Suzanne B. Jordan, "That Lean and Hungry Look," *Newsweek,* October 9, 1978. Reprinted by permission.

4. E. A. H. Sims *et al.*, "Endocrine and Metabolic Effects of Experimental Obesity in Man," *Recent Progress in Hormone Research* 29 (1973): 457.

5. Jerome L. Knittle *et al.*, "The Growth of Adipose Tissue in Children and Adolescents," *Journal of Clinical Investigation* 63 (1979): 239.

6. Robert G. Campbell *et al.*, "Studies of Food-Intake Regulation in Man," *New England Journal of Medicine* 285 (1971): 1402.

7. Ronald J. Dorris and Albert J. Stunkard, "Physical Activity: Performance and Attitudes of a Group of Obese Women," *American Journal of the Medical Sciences* 233 (1957), 622–28.

8. B. A. Bullen *et al.*, "Physical Activity of Obese and Nonobese Adolescent Girls Appraised by Motion Picture Sampling," *American Journal of Clinical Nutrition* 14 (1964): 211.

9. Victor Vertes, "Obesity—A New Approach to an Old Problem," *Heart and Lung* 9 (1980): 719.

10. Albert J. Stunkard *et al.*, "Controlled Trial of Behavior Therapy," *Lancet,* October 15, 1980, pp. 1045–47.

11. S. B. Hulley and S. P. Fortmann, "Clinical Trials of Changing Behavior to Prevent Cardiovascular Disease," in Weiss and Fox, eds., *Perspectives on Behavioral Medicine* 89–98 (1981).

CHAPTER 7

1. James M. Falko *et al.*, "Improvement of High-Density Lipoprotein-Cholesterol Levels," *Journal of the American Medical Association* 247 (1982): 37–39.

2. William B. Kannel and Daniel L. McGee, "Diabetes and Cardiovascular Disease," *Journal of the American Medical Association* 241 (1979): 2035–38.

CHAPTER 8

1. J. N. Morris *et al.*, "Vigorous Exercise in Leisure Time," *Lancet,* December 6, 1980, pp. 1207–10.

2. Antony W. Sedgwick *et al.*, "Long-Term Effects of Physical Training Programme," *British Medical Journal,* July 5, 1980, pp. 7–10.

3. R. S. Paffenbarger, Jr., A. L. Wing, and R. T. Hyde, "Physical Activity as an Index of Heart Attack Risk in College Alumni," *American Journal of Epidemiology* 108 (1978): 161–75.

4. J. L. Boyer and F. W. Kasch, "Exercise Therapy in Hypertensive Men," *Journal of the American Medical Association* 211 (1970): 1658–71; G. Choquette and R. J. Ferguson, "Blood Pressure Reduction in 'Borderline' Hypertensives Following Physical Training," *Canadian Medical Association Journal* 108 (1973): 699–703; J. A. Bonanno and J. D. Lies, "Effect of Physical Training on Coronary Risk Factors," *American Journal of Cardiology* 33 (1979): 760; M. Krotkiewski *et al.*, "Effects of Long-term Physical Training on Body, Fat, Metabolism, and Blood Pressure in Obesity," *Metabolism* 67 (1979): 650–58; O. Roman *et al.*, "Physical Training Program in Arterial Hypertension: A Long-term Prospective Follow-up," *American Journal of Cardiology* 67 (1981): 230–43.

5. R. S. Eliot, "Techniques that can Help You and Your Patients," *Consultant,* February 1982, p. 92.

CHAPTER 9

1. Herbert Benson, *The Relaxation Response.* New York: Avon Books, 1976, p. 59.

2. William Osler, "Lectures on Angina Pectoris and Allied States," *New York Medical Journal* 64 (1896): 177–82.

3. Meyer Friedman and Ray Rosenman, *Type A Behavior and Your Heart.* New York: Alfred A. Knopf, 1974, p. 80.

4. Suzanne G. Haynes *et al.*, "The Relationship of Psychological Factors to Coronary Heart Disease," *American Journal of Epidemiology* 111 (1980): 37–58.

5. Friedman and Rosenman, *op. cit.,* p. 180.

6. R. S. Eliot, "Techniques that can Help You and Your Patients," *Consultant,* February 1982, p. 100.

7. Chandra Patel *et al.*, "Controlled Trial of Biofeedback-Aided Behavioral Methods in Reducing Mild Hypertension," *British Medical Journal* 282 (1981): 2005–8.

CHAPTER 10

1. M. G. Marmot *et al.*, "Alcohol and Mortality: A U-Shaped Curve," *Lancet,* March 14, 1981, pp. 580–83.

2. Ronald E. LaPorte *et al.*, "The Relationship of Alcohol Consumption to Atherosclerotic Heart Disease," *Preventive Medicine* 9 (1980): 22–40.

3. Harvey W. Gruchow and Erica W. Levin, "Drinking Patterns and Coronary Occlusion," *Hospital Physician* (Primary Cardiology Supplement), November 1981, pp. 61–69.

4. W. P. Castelli, "How Many Drinks a Day." *Journal of the American Medical Association,* Nov. 2, 1979, p. 2000.

CHAPTER 11

1. National Center for Health Statistics, U.S. Public Health Service.

2. L. Rosenberg *et al.,* "Myocardial Infarction and Estrogen Therapy in Postmenopausal Women," *New England Journal of Medicine* 294 (1976): 1256.

3. J. D. Shelton, "Prostacyclin from the Uterus and Woman's Cardiovascular Advantage," *Prostaglandins and Medicine* 8 (1982): 459–66.

4. R. I. Pfeffer *et al.,* "Coronary Risk and Estrogen Use in Post-menopausal Women," *American Journal of Epidemiology* 102 (1978): 479; C. Bain *et al.,* "Use of Postmenopausal Hormones and Risk of Myocardial Infarction," *Circulation* 64 (1981): 42; L. Rosenberg *et al.,* "Early Menopause and the Risk of Myocardial Infarction," *American Journal of Obstetrics and Gynecology* 139 (1981): 47; R. K. Ross *et al.,* "Menopausal Oestrogen Therapy and Protection from Death from Ischaemic Heart Disease," *Lancet* 1 (1981): 858–60.

Guide to Further Reading

You may want more information than is provided in this book or to examine some of the original sources for more details. The following books and articles have been selected as current and authoritative.

INTRODUCTION

Belloc, Nedra B., and Breslow, Lester. "Relationship of Physical Health Status and Health Practices." *Preventive Medicine* 1 (1972): 409–21.

U.S. Department of Health, Education, and Welfare. "Healthy People: The Surgeon General's Report on Health Promotion and Disease Prevention." DHEW (PHS) Publication no. 79–55071. Washington, D.C.: 1979.

CHAPTER 1

Byington, Robert; Dyer, Alan R.; Garside, Dan; Liu, Kiang; Moss, Dorothy; Stamler, Jeremiah; and Tsong, Yi: "Recent Trends of Major Coronary Risk Factors in the United States and Other Industrialized Countries." Proceedings of the Conference on Coronary Heart Disease Mortality. U.S. Department of Health, Education, and Welfare. DHEW (PHS) Publication no. 79–1610. Washington, D.C.: 1979, pp. 340–80.

Conolly, Daniel C.; Oxman, Herbert A.; Nobrega, Fred T.; Kurland, Leonard T.; Kennedy, Margaret A.; and Elveback, Lila R. "Coronary Heart Disease in Residents of Rochester, Minnesota, 1950–1975." *Mayo Clinic Proceedings* 56 (1981): 661–72.

Farquhar, John W. *The American Way of Life Need Not Be Hazardous to Your Health.* New York: 1978, W. W. Norton & Co.

Fries, James F. "Aging, Natural Death, and the Compression of Morbidity." *New England Journal of Medicine* 303 (1980): 130–35.

Gori, G. B., and Richter, B. J. "Macroeconomics of Disease Prevention in the United States." *Science* 200 (1978): 1126.

Levy, Robert I. "Declining Mortality in Coronary Heart Disease." *Arteriosclerosis* 1 (1981): 312–25.

CHAPTER 2

American Heart Association, AHA Committee Report: "Risk Factors and Coronary Disease." Vol. 62, no. 2 (1980): 449A–455A.

Dawber, Thomas Royle. *The Framingham Study: The Epidemiology of Atherosclerotic Disease.* Cambridge: Harvard University Press, 1980.

Hopkins, Paul N., and Williams, Roger R. "A Survey of 246 Suggested Coronary Risk Factors." *Atherosclerosis* 40 (1981): 1–52.

Keys, Ancel. *Seven Countries: A Multivariate Analysis of Death and Coronary Heart Disease.* Cambridge: Harvard University Press, 1980.

Khosla, T.; Newcombe, R. G.; and Campbell, H. "Who Is at Risk of a Coronary?" *British Medical Journal* 1 (1977): 341–44.

Rose, Geoffrey. "Strategy of Prevention: Lessons from Cardiovascular Disease." *British Medical Journal* 282 (1981): 1847–51.

CHAPTER 3

Castelli, William P.; Dawber, Thomas R.; Feinleib, Manning; Garrison, Robert J.; McNamara, Patricia M.; Kannel, William B. "The Filter Cigarette and Coronary Heart Disease: The Framingham Study." *Lancet,* July 18, 1981, pp. 109–13.

Evans, Richard I.; Rozelle, Richard M.; Mittlemark, Maurice B.; Hansen, William B.; Bane, Alice L.; and Havis, Janet. "Deterring the Onset of Smoking in Children: Knowledge of Immediate Physiological Effects and Coping with Peer Pressure, Media Pressure, and Parent Modeling." *Journal of Applied Social Psychology* 8 (1978): 126–35.

Friedman, Gary D.; Dales, Loring G.; and Ury, Hans K. "Mortality in Middle-Aged Smokers and Nonsmokers." *New England Journal of Medicine* 300 (1979): 213–17.

Gordon, Tavia; Kannel, William B.; and McGee, Daniel. "Death and Coronary Attacks in Men after Giving Up Cigarette Smoking: A Report from the Framingham Study." *Lancet,* December 7, 1974, pp. 1345–48.

Gyntelberg, Finn; Pedersen, Peter Beck; Lauridsen, Lone; Schubell, Ken. "Smoking and Risk of Myocardial Infarction in Copenhagen Men Aged 40–59 with Special Reference to Cheroot Smoking." *Lancet,* May 2, 1981, pp. 987–89.

Kannel, William B. "Update on the Role of Cigarette Smoking in Coronary Artery Disease." *American Heart Journal* 101, no. 3 (1981): 319–28.

Lando, Harry A. "Successful Treatment of Smokers with a Broad-Spectrum Behavioral Approach." *Journal of Consulting and Clinical Psychology* 45 (1977): 361–66.

Rose, Geoffrey, and Hamilton, P.J.S. "A Randomized Controlled Trial of the Effect on Middle-Aged Men of Advice to Stop Smoking." *Journal of Epidemiology and Community Health* 32 (1978): 275–81.

Sobel, Robert. *They Satisfy.* New York: Anchor Press/Doubleday, 1978.

Wald, Nicholas J.; Idle, Marianne; Boreham, Jillian; Bailey, Alan; and Van Vunakis, Helen. "Serum Continine Levels in Pipe Smokers: Evidence against Nicotine as Cause of Coronary Heart Disease." *Lancet,* October 10, 1981, pp. 775–77.

CHAPTER 4

Guttmacher, Sally; Teitelman, Michael; Chapin, Georganne; Gabrowski, Gail; and Schnall, Peter. "Ethics and Preventive Medicine: The Case of Borderline Hypertension." Hastings Center Report, February, 1981, pp. 12–20.

Hypertension Detection and Follow-Up Program Cooperative Group. "Reduction in Mortality of Persons with High Blood Pressure, Including Mild Hypertension." *Journal of the American Medical Association* 243 (1979): 2562–71.

Joint National Committee on Detection, Evaluation, and Treatment of High Blood Pressure. "The 1980 Report of the Joint National Committee on Detection, Evaluation, and Treatment of High Blood Pressure." *Archives of Internal Medicine* 140 (1980): 1280–84.

Kaplan, N. M. *Clinical Hypertension.* 3d ed. Baltimore: Williams and Williams, 1982.

Kerr, C. M.; Reisinger, K. S.; and Plankey, F. W. "Sodium Concentration of Homemade Baby Foods." *Pediatrics* 63 (1978): 331–35.

Management Committee. "The Australian Therapeutic Trial in Mild Hypertension." *Lancet* 2 (1980): 1261–67.

Ram, C. Venkata S.; Garrett, Bruce N.; and Kaplan, Norman M. "Moderate Sodium Restriction and Various Diuretics in the Treatment of Hypertension." *Archives of Internal Medicine* 141 (1981): 1015–19.

Society of Actuaries and Association of Life Insurance Medical Directors of America. "Blood Pressure Study, 1979." November, 1980.

Stamler, Jeremiah; Farinaro, Eduardo; Mojonnier, Louise M.; Hall, Yolanda; Moss, Dorothy; and Stamler, Rose. "Prevention and Control of Hypertension by Nutritional-Hygienic Means." *Journal of the American Medical Association* 243 (1980): 1819–23.

Tuck, Michael L.; Sowers, James; Dornfeld, Leslie; Kledzik, Gary; and Maxwell, Morton. "The Effect of Weight Reduction on Blood Pressure, Plasma Renin Activity, and Plasma Aldosterone Levels in Obese Patients." *New England Journal of Medicine* 304 (1981): 930–33.

VA Cooperative Study Group on Antihypertensive Agents. "Effects of Treatment on Morbidity in Hypertension. III. Influence of Age, Diastolic Pressure and Prior Cardiovascular Disease. Further Analysis of Side Effects." *Circulation* 45 (1972): 441.

CHAPTER 5

Bordia, Arun. "Effects of Garlic on Blood Lipids in Patients with Coronary Heart Disease." *American Journal of Clinical Nutrition* 34 (1981): 2100–3.

Hjermann, I.; Holme, I.; Velve Byre, K.; and Leren, P. "Effect of Diet and Smoking Intervention on the Incidence of Coronary Heart Disease." *Lancet* 2 (1981): 1303–10.

Oliver, M. F. "Diet and Coronary Heart Disease." *British Medical Bulletin* 37 (1981): 49–58.

Roberts, Susan L.; McMurry, Martha P.; and Connor, William E. "Does Egg Feeding [i.e., dietary cholesterol] Affect Plasma Cholesterol Levels in Humans? The Results of a Double-Blind Study." *American Journal of Clinical Nutrition* 34 (1981): 2092–99.

Stamler, Jeremiah. "Population Studies" in *Nutrition, Lipids and Coronary Heart Disease*. Edited by R. I. Levy; B. Rifkind; B. Dennis; and N. Ernst. New York: Raven Press, 1979, pp. 25–88.

Voller, Robert D., and Strong, William B. "Pediatric Aspects of Atherosclerosis." *American Heart Journal* 101 (1981): 815–36.

CHAPTER 6

Campbell, Robert G.; Hashim, Sami A.; and Van Itallie, Theodore B. "Studies of Food-Intake Regulation in Man." *New England Journal of Medicine* 285 (1971): 1402–5.

Coates, Thomas J.; Jeffery, Robert W.; and Slinkard, Lee Ann. "Heart Healthy Eating and Exercise: Introducing and Maintaining Changes in Health Behaviors." *American Journal of Public Health* 71 (1981): 15–23.

Drenick, Ernst J.; Bale, Gurunanjappa S.; Seltzer, Frederic; and Johnson, Daisie G. "Excessive Mortality and Causes of Death in Morbidly Obese Men." *Journal of the American Heart Association* 243 (1980): 443–45.

Fitzgerald, Faith T. "The Problem of Obesity." *Annual Review of Medicine* 32 (1981): 221–31.

Himes, John H. "Infant Feeding Practices and Obesity." *Journal of the American Dietetic Association* 75 (1979): 122–25.

Isner, Jeffrey M.; Sours, Harold E.; Paris, Allen L.; Ferrans, Victor J.; and Roberts, William C. "Sudden, Unexpected Death in Avid Dieters Using the Liquid-Protein-Modified-Fast Diet." *Circulation* 60 (1979): 1401–12.

Johnson, M. L.; Burke, Bertha S.; and Mayer, J. "Relative Importance of Inactivity and Overeating in the Energy Balance of Obese High School Girls." *American Journal of Clinical Nutrition* 4 (1956): 37–54.

Keys, Ancel. "Overweight, Obesity, Coronary Heart Disease and Mortality." *Nutrition Reviews* 38 (1980): 297–307.

Knittle, J. L., and Hirsch, J. "Effect of Early Nutrition on the Development of Rat Epididymal Fat Pads." *Journal of Clinical Investigation* 47 (1968): 2091.

Knittle, J. L.; Timmers, Kim; Ginsberg-Fellner, Fredda; Brown, Roy E.; and Katz, David P. "The Growth of Adipose Tissue in Children and Adolescents." *Journal of Clinical Investigation* 63 (1979): 239–46.

Kuller, Lewis H.; Crook, Marie; Almes, Mary Jane; Detre, Katherine; Reese, Grace; and Rutan, Gale. "Dormont High School [Pittsburgh, Pennsylvania] Blood Pressure Study." *Hypertension* 2, supplement 1 (1980): 109–16.

Sims, Ethan A. H., and Berchtold, Peter. "Obesity and Hypertension." *Journal of the American Medical Association* 247 (1982): 49–52.

Sorlie, Paul; Gordon, Tavia; and Kannel, William B. "Body Build and Mortality." *Journal of the American Medical Associatian* 243 (1980): 1828–31.

Stunkard, Albert J.; O'Brien, Richard; and Craighead, Linda Wilcoxon. "Controlled Trial of Behaviour Therapy, Pharmacotherapy, and Their Combination in the Treatment of Obesity." *Lancet*, October 15, 1980, pp. 1045–47.

Vertes, Victor. "Obesity—A New Approach to an Old Problem." *Heart and Lung* 9 (1980): 719–25.

CHAPTER 7

Falko, James M.; O'Dorisio, M.; and Cataland, Samuel. "Improvement of High-Density Lipoprotein-Cholesterol Levels." *Journal of the American Medical Association* 247 (1982): 37–39.

Fuller, John H.; Shipley, Martin J.; Rose, Geoffrey; Jarrett, John R.; and Keen, Harry. "Coronary-Heart-Disease Risk and Impaired Glucose Tolerance." *Lancet* 1 (1980): 1373–76.

Kannel, William B.; and McGee, Daniel L. "Diabetes and Cardiovascular Disease." *Journal of the American Medical Association* 241 (1979):2035–38.

National Diabetes Data Group. "Classification and Diagnosis of Diabetes Mellitus and Other Categories of Glucose Intolerance." *Diabetes* 28 (1979): 1039–57.

CHAPTER 8

American College of Sports Medicine. "The Recommended Quantity and Quality of Exercise for Developing and Maintaining Fitness in Healthy Adults." *Medicine and Science in Sports* 10 (1978): vii–x.

Blumenthal, James A.; Williams, R. Sanders; Williams, Redford B., Jr.; and Wallace, Andrew G. "Effects of Exercise on the Type A [coronary prone] Behavior Pattern." *Psychosomatic Medicine* 43 (1980): 289–95.

Brand, Richard J.; Paffenbarger, Ralph S., Jr.; Sholtz, Robert I.; and Kampert, James B. "Work Activity and Fatal Heart Attack Studied by Multiple Logistic Risk Analysis." *American Journal of Epidemiology* 110 (1979): 52–62.

Carr, Daniel B.; Bullen, Beverly A.; Skrinar, Gary S.; Arnold, Michael A.; Rosenblatt, Michael; Beitins, Inese Z.; Martin, Joseph B.; and McArthur, Janet W. "Physical Conditioning Facilitates the Exercise-Induced Secretion of Beta-Endorphin and Beta-Lipotropin in Women." *New England Journal of Medicine* 305 (1981): 560–62.

Ewing, D. J.; Irving, J. B.; Kerr, F.; and Kirby, Brian J. "Static Exercise in Untreated Systemic Hypertension." *British Heart Journal* 35 (1973): 413–21.

Franklin, Barry A., and Rubenfire, Melvyn. "Losing Weight through Exercise." *Journal of the American Medical Association* 244 (1980): 377–79.

Hartung, G. Harley; Foreyt, John P.; Mitchell, Robert E.; Vlasek, Imogene; and Gotto, Antonio M., Jr. "Relation of Diet to High-Density-Lipoprotein Cholesterol in Middle-Aged Marathon Runners, Joggers, and Inactive Men." *New England Journal of Medicine* 302 (1980): 356–61.

Huttunen, Jussi K.; Länsimies, Esko; Voutilainen, Erkki; Enholm, Christian; Hietanen, Eino; Penttilä, Ilkka; Siitonen, Onni; and Rauramaa, Rainer. "Effect of Moderate Physical Exercise on Serum Lipoproteins." *Circulation* 60 (1979): 1220–29.

Kramsch, Dieter M.; Aspen, Anita J.; Abramowitz, Bruce M.; Kreimendahl, Toby; and Hood, William B., Jr.; "Reduction of Coronary Atherosclerosis by Moderate Conditioning Exercise in Monkeys on an Atherogenic Diet." *New England Journal of Medicine* 305 (1981): 1483–89.

Morris, J. N.; Pollard, R.; Everitt, M. G.; Chave, S. P. W. "Vigorous

Exercise in Leisure Time: Protection against Coronary Heart Disease." *Lancet,* December 6, 1980, pp. 1207–10.

Sedgwick, Antony W.; Brotherhood, John R.; Harris-Davidson, Ann; Taplin, Roger E.; and Thomas, David W. "Long-Term Effects of Physical Training Programme on Risk Factors for Coronary Heart Disease in Otherwise Sedentary Men." *British Medical Journal,* July 5, 1980, pp. 7–10.

CHAPTER 9

Berkman, Lisa F.; and Syme, S. Leonard. "Social Networks, Host Resistance, and Mortality: A Nine-Year Follow-Up Study of Alameda County Residents." *American Journal of Epidemiology* 109 (1979): 186–204.

Brand, Richard J.; Rosenman, Ray H.; Sholtz, Robert I.; and Friedman, Meyer. "Multivariate Prediction of Coronary Heart Disease in the Western Collaborative Group Study Compared to the Findings of the Framingham Study." *Circulation* 53 (1976): 348–55.

Friedman, Meyer, and Rosenman, Ray H. *Type A Behavior and Your Heart.* New York: Alfred A. Knopf, 1974.

Haynes, Suzanne G.; Feinleib, Manning; and Kannel, William. "The Relationship of Psychosocial Factors to Coronary Heart Disease in the Framingham Study." *American Journal of Epidemiology* 111 (1980): 37–58.

Herman, Steve; Blumenthal, James A.; Black, George M.; and Chesney, Margaret A. "Self-Ratings of Type A [Coronary Prone] Adults: Do Type A's Know They Are Type A's?" *Psychosomatic Medicine* 43 (1981): 405–13.

Patel, Chandra; Marmot, M. G.; and Terry, D. J. "Controlled Trial of Biofeedback-Aided Behavioural Methods in Reducing Mild Hypertension." *British Medical Journal* 282 (1981): 2005–8.

Review Panel on Coronary-Prone Behavior and Coronary Heart Disease. "Coronary-Prone Behavior and Coronary Heart Disease: A Critical Review." *Circulation* 63 (1981): 1199–1215.

Rose, Geoffrey, and Marmot, M. G. "Social Class and Coronary Heart Disease." *American Heart Journal* 45 (1981): 13–19.

CHAPTER 10

Celentano, David D.; Martines, Rose Marie; and McQueen, David V. "The Association of Alcohol Consumption and Hypertension." *Preventive Medicine* 10 (1981): 590–602.

Gordon, Tavia; Ernst, Nancy; Fisher, Marian; and Rifkind, Basil M. "Alcohol and High-Density Lipoprotein Cholesterol." *Circulation* 64 supp. 3 (1981): 63–76.

Gruchow, Harvey W., and Levin, Erica Wexman. "Drinking Patterns and Coronary Occlusion." *Hospital Physician* (Primary Cardiology Supplement), November, 1981, pp. 61–69.

Eckardt, Michael J.; Hartford, Thomas C.; Kaelber, Charles T.; Parker, Elizabeth S.; Rosenthal, Laura S.; Ryback, Ralph S.; Salmoiraghi, Gian C.; Vanderveen, Ernestine; and Warren, Kenneth R. "Health Hazards Associated with Alcohol Consumption." *Journal of the American Medical Association* 246 (1981): 648–66.

Klatsky, Arthur L.; Friedman, Gary D.; and Siegelaub, Abraham B. "Alcohol and Mortality." *Annals of Internal Medicine* 95 (1981): 139–45.

LaPorte, Ronald E.; Cresanta, James L.; and Kuller, Lewis H. "The Relationship of Alcohol Consumption to Atherosclerotic Heart Disease." *Preventive Medicine* 9 (1980): 22–40.

Marmot, M. G.; Shipley, M. J.; Rose, Geoffrey; and Thomas, Briony J. "Alcohol and Mortality: A U-Shaped Curve." *Lancet,* March 14, 1981, pp. 580–83.

Yano, Katsuhiko; Rhoads, George G.; and Kagan, Abraham. "Coffee, Alcohol and Risk of Coronary Heart Disease among Japanese Men Living in Hawaii." *New England Journal of Medicine* 297 (1977): 405–9.

CHAPTER 11

Bain, Christopher; Willett, Walter; Hennekens, Charles H.; Rosner, Bernard; Belanger, Charlene; and Speizer, Frank E. "Use of Postmenopausal Hormones and Risk of Myocardial Infarction." *Circulation* 64 (1981): 42–46.

Centerwall, Brandon S. "Premenopausal Hysterectomy and Cardiovascular Disease." *American Journal of Obstetrics and Gynecology* 139 (1981): 58–61.

Gordon, Tavia; Kannel, William B.; Hjortland, Marthana C.; and McNamara, Patricia M. "Menopause and Coronary Heart Disease." *Annals of Internal Medicine* 89 (1978): 156–61.

Kruegar, Dean E. *et al.* "Risk Factors for Fatal Heart Attack in Young Women." *American Journal of Epidemiology* 113 (1981): 357–70.

Rosenberg, Lynn; Slone, Dennis; Shapiro, Samuel; Kaufman, David; Stolley, Paul; and Miettinen, Olli S. "Noncontraceptive Estrogens and Myocardial Infarction in Young Women," *Journal of the American Medical Association* 244 (1980): 339–42.

Walker, Alexander M. *et al.* "Vasectomy and Non-Fatal Myocardial Infarction." *Lancet,* January 3, 1981, pp. 13–15.

CHAPTER 12

Canadian Cooperative Study Group. "A Randomized Trial of Aspirin and Sulfinpyrazone in Threatened Stroke." *New England Journal of Medicine* 299 (1978): 53–59.

Genton, Edward. "A Perspective on Platelet-Suppressant Drug Treatment in Coronary Artery and Cerebrovascular Disease." *Circulation* 62, supp. 5 (1980): 111–21.

Hedstrand, H., and Aberg, H. "Familial History in Males at Low and High Risk for Cardiovascular Disease." *Preventive Medicine* 7 (1978): 15–21.

Heyden, Siegfried; Tyroler, Herman A.; Heiss, Gerardo; Hames, Curtis G.; and Bartel, Alan. "Coffee Consumption and Mortality." *Archives of Internal Medicine* 138 (1978): 1472–75.

Hirsh, Paul D.; Campbell, William B.; Willerson, James T.; and Hillis, David L. "Prostaglandins and Ischemic Heart Disease." *American Journal of Medicine* 71 (1981): 1099–1126.

Wu, Kenneth K. *et al.* "Differential Effects of Two Doses of Aspirin on Platelet-Vessel Wall Interaction in Vivo." *Journal of Clinical Investigation* 68 (1981): 382–87.

Index

circulation, in normal heart, 12–
16
coarctation of aorta, and hypertension, 60
colon cancer, dietary fiber and,
88
congestive heart failure, hypertension and, 57–58
cooking
lower fat diet and, 83, 87
low-sodium, 63
coronary arteries, 15
See also coronary heart
disease
coronary blood vessels, 157
narrowing, and drinking behavior, 157
Coronary Care Unit (CCU), 19
coronary heart disease, 4, 16–18
death rates from, 77
moderate alcohol intake and
risk reduction for, 151–58
obesity and, 94
socioeconomic class and,
143–45
See also heart disease
coronary thrombosis, 18
Cushing's disease, hypertension
and, 60

death rates. See mortality rates
from cardiovascular disease
diabetes, 22
blood sugar levels and vascular disease, 121–22
as cardiovascular disease risk
factor, 24–25
classifications, 119–20

management of, 121–22
obesity and, 94–95
risks of, 118–22
vascular disease and, 120–21
diastolic pressure, 14, 50, 51
diet
blood cholesterol levels and,
9, 10
changes in, 6
diabetes and, 120, 121
in "Diet-Heart" model, 78–
79, 80
fiber in, 88–89
hypertension and, 61
low-fat, 90–91
lower-fat, 82–89
sodium in, 53–56
sodium-restricted, 62–70
diet pills, and antihypertensives,
72
diet programs, 108–9, 111
fad diets, 9, 11, 105–6
disease predictors. See risk
factors
disease prevention, health practices and, viii–ix
diuretic drugs, 54–55
hypertension and, 72–74
drugs
dependence on, 34–35
for hypertension, 60, 70–74
See also specific names

edema, hypertension and, 57–58
educational programs
infant feeding and, 31
in nutrition, 117
egg yolks, 83, 87